MEDICAL
TERMINOLOGY:

A
SHORT
COURSE

MEDICAL TERMINOLOGY:

A SHORT COURSE

DAVI-ELLEN CHABNER, B.A., M.A.T.

1991

W.B. SAUNDERS COMPANY
Harcourt Brace Jovanovich, Inc.

Philadelphia · *London* · *Toronto* · *Montreal* · *Sydney* · *Tokyo*

W. B. SAUNDERS COMPANY
Harcourt Brace Jovanovich, Inc.

The Curtis Center
Independence Square West
Philadelphia, PA 19106

Library of Congress Cataloging-in-Publication Data

Chabner, Davi-Ellen.
    Medical terminology : a short course / Davi-Ellen Chabner.
       p. cm.
    ISBN 0-7216-2939-3
    1. Medicine — Terminology.   I. Title.
    [DNLM: 1. Nomenclature.   W 15 C427m]
    R123.C434 1991
    616′.0014 — dc20
    DNLM/DLC
    for Library of Congress   90-8177
                                              CIP

Editor: Margaret M. Biblis

Developmental Editor: Leslie E. Hoeltzel

Manuscript Editor: Donna Walker

Designer: Joan Sinclair

Production Manager: Frank Polizzano

To my family and my friends
for their unwavering support, encouragement, and love
and
To Howie
for his devoted companionship and loyalty

PREFACE

This text is intended for use in a short course of medical terminology, from 12 to 20 hours. During the past several years, I have been teaching this course in hospitals and to groups from health maintenance organizations, adult education programs, insurance companies, and other allied health groups. This book began as I saw the need for a teaching text to use with my students. It does not aim to present complete instruction in medical terminology; rather, its goal is to give an introduction and overview, with emphasis on basic, practical terms. In addition, its illustrations and ample appendices and glossaries are designed to serve as important references long after the short course is completed.

Here are some of the features of the book:

1. It is a *workbook-text format,* following the teaching method in my longer, more complete text, *The Language of Medicine.* You will learn by doing; that is, by writing answers to exercises, labeling diagrams, testing yourself with review sheets, and saying terms out loud while following pronunciation guides in each chapter.

2. It is *visual,* including many line diagrams that illustrate terminology. Each chapter contains simple diagrams that highlight parts of the body, procedures, and even disease conditions. In addition, *Appendix I: Body Systems* is a collection of labeled diagrams of each system of the body that will help you identify and remember terms as you work through the text, and as you encounter terminology in your job.

3. It is *easy to read and understand* because I have not presupposed prior knowledge of science or biology. Explanations of terms are worded simply and clearly, and repetition is used to reinforce understanding all through the text. Answers to each exercise are given directly following the exercise, so that you can conveniently check your response and easily learn from the printed answers.

4. It is a valuable *reference* for your use during and after you complete your termi-

nology course. In addition to the diagrams in Appendix I, *Appendix II: Diagnostic Tests and Procedures* is a list of explanations of clinical procedures and laboratory tests that are helpful to a person working in the allied health field. *Appendix III: Abbreviations and Symbols* lists commonly used medical abbreviations and symbols and their meanings. In addition, all terms in the text are defined in the comprehensive *Glossary of Terms* at the end of the book. Finally, the *Glossary of Word Parts* presents medical terminology word parts (combining forms, suffixes, and prefixes) with their English meanings and then in a separate list reverses the process, giving English words and their Medical Terminology counterparts.

I hope that you enjoy using this text, and appreciate its simplicity and practicality. It is a combination of commonly used terminology and "hands-on" visually reinforced learning designed to introduce the beginning student to the medical language. It will also serve as a useful guide and reference to medical terms long after your formal course has been completed. Most of all, though, I hope that this book excites your interest and enthusiasm for the medical language, making a difference in your work experience, as well as your personal involvement with health issues. I guarantee that, by faithfully working through this book, you can begin to learn the medical language, and its usefulness will help you throughout your life.

Finally, I welcome hearing from you with suggestions and comments, since I am always learning from students and their teachers. Work hard, and have fun with medical terms!

ACKNOWLEDGMENTS

My students at Kaiser Permanente (of the Washington, D.C. area) and at Providence Hospital (Washington, D.C.) deserve the credit for testing this book during many hours of instruction and study. They are my partners in this endeavor, and I hope the final product is useful and helpful to other students of medical terminology.

Bruce Chabner, M.D., Elizabeth Chabner, and Judy McGinnis gave support and advice from conception through production of the book, and I'm grateful for their comments and suggestions.

Special thanks to Maria Christina Osorio for assisting in assembling the index, and to Julia Osorio for taking care of the details of my life, so that I could be free to work.

Finally, much gratitude to the staff at W.B. Saunders for working with me and supporting the project.

CONTENTS

CHAPTER 1

BASIC WORD STRUCTURE

CHAPTER OBJECTIVES

- To divide medical terms into component parts
- To analyze, pronounce, and spell medical terms using common combining forms, suffixes, and prefixes

I. WORD ANALYSIS

If you work in a medical setting, you use medical words every day. As a consumer and citizen, you hear medical terms in your doctor's office, read about health issues in the newspaper, and make daily decisions about your own health care and the health care of your family. Terms such as *arthritis, electrocardiogram, hepatitis,* and *anemia* describe conditions and tests that are familiar. Other medical words are more complicated, but as you work in this book, you will begin to understand them even if you have never studied biology or science.

Medical words are like individual jigsaw puzzles. Once you divide the terms into their component parts and learn the meaning of the individual parts, you can use that knowledge to understand many other new terms.

For example, the term HEMATOLOGY is divided into three parts:

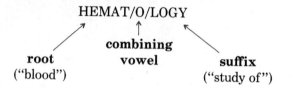

When you analyze a medical term, begin at the *end* of the word. The ending is called a **suffix.** All medical terms contain suffixes. The suffix in HEMATOLOGY is -LOGY, which means "study of." Now look at the beginning of the term. HEMAT is the word **root.** The root gives the essential meaning of the term. The root HEMAT- means "blood."

The third part of this term, which is the letter O, has no meaning of its own but is an important connector between the root (HEMAT) and the suffix (LOGY). It is called a **combining vowel.** The letter O is the combining vowel usually found in medical terms.

Putting together the meaning of the suffix and the root, the term HEMATOLOGY means "the study of blood."

Here's another familiar medical term: ELECTROCARDIOGRAM. You probably know this term, often abbreviated as EKG or ECG. This is how you divide it into its parts:

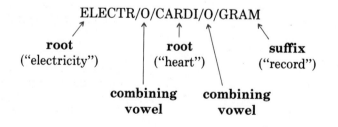

Start with the **suffix** at the end of the term. The suffix -GRAM means "a record."

Now look at the beginning of the term. ELECTR- is a word **root,** and it means "electricity."

This medical term has two roots. The second root is CARDI-, meaning "heart." Whenever you see CARDI in other medical terms, you will know that it means "heart."

Read the meaning of medical terms from the suffix, back to the beginning of the term, then across. Thus, the entire term means "record of the electricity in the heart." It is the electricity flowing within the heart that causes the heart muscle to contract, pumping blood throughout your body. The contraction and relaxation of heart muscle are called the heartbeat.

Notice the two combining vowels in ELECTROCARDIOGRAM. Looking for the O in medical terms will help you divide the term into its parts. A combining vowel (O) lies between roots (ELECTR and CARDI) and between the root (CARDI) and suffix (GRAM).

The combining vowel *plus* the root is called a **combining form.** For example, there are *two* combining forms in the word ELECTROCARDIOGRAM. These combining forms are ELECTR/O, meaning "electricity," and CARDI/O, meaning "heart."

Notice how the following medical term is analyzed. Can you locate the two combining forms in this term?

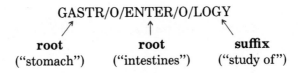

GASTR/O/ENTER/O/LOGY

root	root	suffix
("stomach")	("intestines")	("study of")

The two combining forms are GASTR/O and ENTER/O. The entire word (reading from the suffix, back to the beginning of the term, and across) means "study of the stomach and the intestines." Here are other words that are divided into component parts:

GASTR/O/SCOPE   means   "Instrument to visually examine the stomach."

combining **suffix**
form ("instrument
("stomach") to visually
examine")

GASTR/IC   means   "Pertaining to the stomach." Notice that the combining vowel is *dropped* when the suffix (-IC) begins with a vowel. Words ending in -IC are adjectives and mean "pertaining to."

root **suffix**
("stomach") ("pertaining to")

CARDI/AC   means   "Pertaining to the heart." Again, the combining vowel is dropped when the suffix (-AC) begins with a vowel. Words ending in -AC are adjectives and mean "pertaining to."

root **suffix**
("heart") ("pertaining to")

ENTER/ITIS   means   "Inflammation of the intestines." Notice again that the combining vowel is dropped because the suffix (-ITIS) begins with a vowel.

root **suffix**
("intestines") ("inflammation")

GASTR/O/ENTER/ITIS means   "Inflammation of the stomach and intestines." Notice
that the combining vowel (O) remains between the two
roots even though the second root (ENTER) begins
with a vowel.

root | **suffix**
("stomach") | ("inflammation")

root
("intestines")

In addition to roots, suffixes, combining forms, and combining vowels, many medical terms have a word part attached to the *beginning* of the term. This is called a **prefix,** and it can change the meaning of a term in important ways. For example, watch what happens to the meaning of the following medical terms when the prefix changes:

SUB/gastr/ic   means   "pertaining to *below* the stomach."

prefix
("below")

TRANS/gastr/ic   means   "pertaining to *across* the stomach."

prefix
("across")

RETRO/gastr/ic   means   "pertaining to *behind* the stomach."

prefix
("behind")

Let's **review** the important word parts:

1. **Root** — gives the essential *meaning* of the term.
2. **Suffix** — is the word *ending.*
3. **Prefix** — is a small part added to the *beginning* of a term.
4. **Combining vowel** — *connects* roots to suffixes and roots to other roots.
5. **Combining form** — is the combination of the *root* and *combining vowel.*

Some important rules to *remember* are:

1. *Read* the meaning of medical words from the suffix to the beginning of the word and then across.
2. *Drop* the combining vowel before a suffix that starts with a vowel.
3. *Keep* the combining vowel between word roots, even if the root begins with a vowel.

II. COMBINING FORMS, SUFFIXES, AND PREFIXES

Here is a list of combining forms, suffixes, and prefixes that are commonly found in medical terms. Write the meaning of the medical term on the line that is provided. As you study medical terminology, you will find it helpful to practice writing terms and their meanings many times. Complete the *exercises* in Section III, the *review* in Section IV, and the *pronunciation of terms* list in Section V, and you will have begun your study of medical language.

Combining Forms

Combining Form	Meaning	Medical Term	Meaning
aden/o	gland	adenoma _____ -OMA means "tumor" or "mass."	
		adenitis _____ -ITIS means "inflammation."	
arthr/o	joint	arthritis _____	
bi/o	life	biology _____ -LOGY means "study of."	
		biopsy _____ -OPSY means "to view." Living tissue is removed and viewed under a microscope.	
carcin/o	cancerous	carcinoma _____	
cardi/o	heart	cardiology _____	
cephal/o	head	cephalic _____ -IC means "pertaining to."	
cerebr/o	cerebrum, largest part of the brain	cerebral _____ -AL means "pertaining to." Figure 1–1 shows the cerebrum and some of its functions.	
		cerebrovascular accident (CVA) _____ -VASCULAR means "pertaining to blood vessels"; a CVA is commonly known as a stroke.	
cyst/o	urinary bladder	cystoscope _____ -SCOPE means "instrument to visually examine." Figure 1–2 shows the urinary tract. A cystoscope is placed through the urethra into the urinary bladder.	
cyt/o	cell	cytology _____	

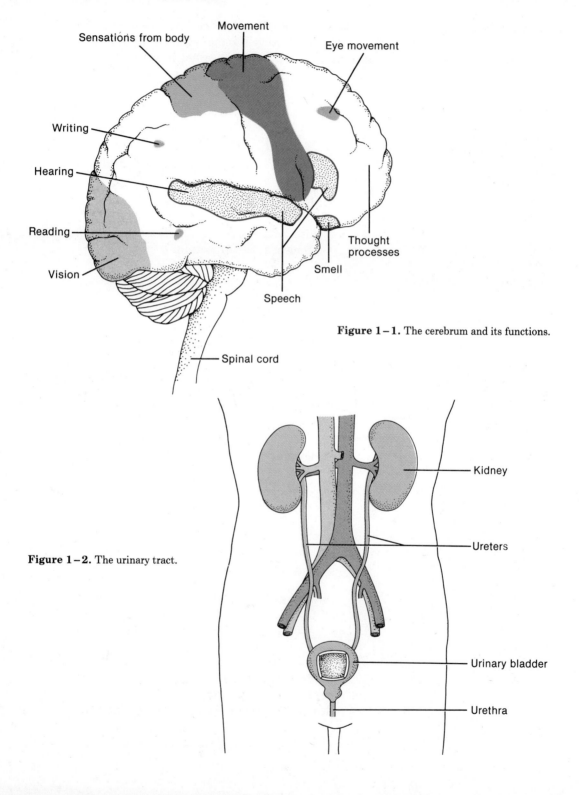

Figure 1–1. The cerebrum and its functions.

Figure 1–2. The urinary tract.

dermat/o	skin
electr/o	electricity
encephal/o	brain
enter/o	intestines (often the small intestine)

dermatitis _____

electrocardiogram (ECG, EKG) _____
-GRAM means "record."

electroencephalogram (EEG) _____

enteritis _____
Figure 1–3 shows the small and large intestines. ENTER/O is used to describe the small intestine and the intestines in general, while COL/O is the combining form for the large intestine (colon).

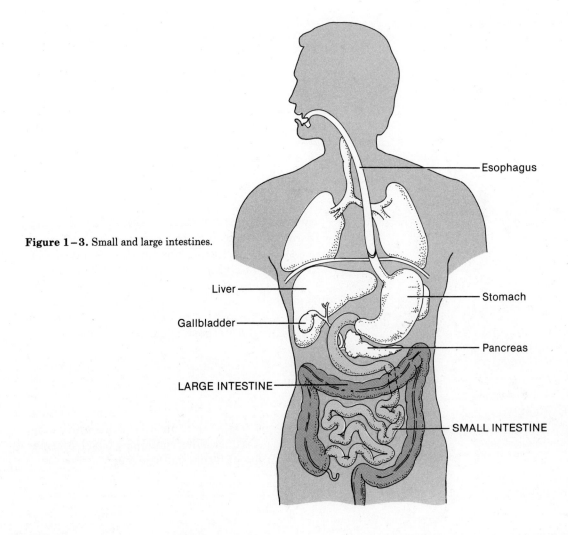

Figure 1–3. Small and large intestines.

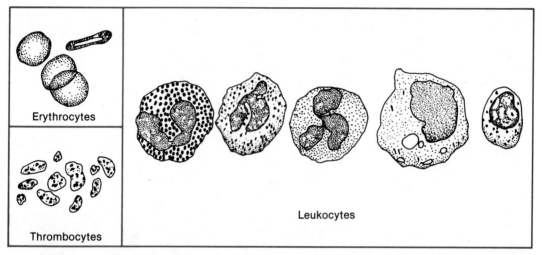

Figure 1-4. Blood cells: erythrocytes (carry oxygen), leukocytes (five different types help fight disease), and thrombocytes or platelets (help blood to clot).

erythr/o	red

erythrocyte _____
-CYTE means "cell." Figure 1-4 shows the three major types of blood cells.

gastr/o	stomach

gastroscopy _____
-SCOPY means "process of viewing."

gnos/o	knowledge

diagnosis _____
-SIS means "state of"; DIA- means "complete." A diagnosis is the complete knowledge that is gained after testing and examining the patient.

prognosis _____
PRO- means "before." A prognosis is a prediction that is made after the diagnosis about the outcome of treatment.

gynec/o	woman

gynecology _____

hemat/o	blood

hematoma _____
-OMA means "mass" or "tumor." In this term, -oma indicates a mass or swelling containing blood. A hematoma is a bruise or black-and-blue mark.

hepat/o	liver

hepatitis _____

lapar/o	abdomen (area between the chest and hip)

laparotomy _____
-TOMY means "incision" (to cut into). An exploratory laparotomy is an incision of the abdominal wall to inspect abdominal organs for evidence of disease.

leuk/o	white

leukocyte _____
Figure 1–4 shows leukocytes.

nephr/o	kidney

nephrectomy _____
-ECTOMY means "to cut out," an excision or resection of an organ or part of the body.

neur/o	nerve

neurology _____

oste/o	bone

osteoarthritis _____
Figure 1–5 shows a normal joint and a joint with osteoarthritis.

onc/o	tumor

oncologist _____
-IST means "a specialist."

ophthalm/o	eye

ophthalmoscope _____

path/o	disease

pathologist _____
A pathologist is a medical doctor who views biopsy samples to make a diagnosis and examines a dead body (autopsy) to determine the cause of death. AUT- means "self" and -OPSY means "to view." Thus, an autopsy is an opportunity to see for oneself what has happened to the patient to cause his or her death.

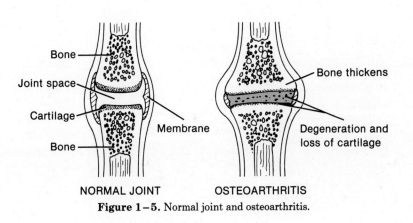

NORMAL JOINT   OSTEOARTHRITIS

Figure 1–5. Normal joint and osteoarthritis.

psych/o	mind	psychosis _____
		-OSIS means "abnormal condition." This is a serious mental condition in which the patient loses touch with reality.
ren/o	kidney	renal _____
		Sometimes there are *two* combining forms for the same part of the body. One comes from Latin, and the other from Greek (REN- is the Latin root meaning "kidney," and NEPHR- is the Greek root). The Greek root is used to describe abnormal conditions and procedures, whereas the Latin root is used with -AL, meaning "pertaining to."
rhin/o	nose	rhinitis _____
sarc/o	flesh	sarcoma _____
		Sarcomas and carcinomas are cancerous tumors. Sarcomas grow from the "fleshy" tissues of the body, such as muscle, fat, bone, and cartilage, whereas carcinomas arise from skin tissue and the linings of internal organs.
thromb/o	clotting	thrombocyte _____
		A thrombocyte (platelet) is a small cell that helps blood to clot. Platelets are shown in Figure 1–4.
		thrombosis _____
		A thrombus (blood clot) occurs when thrombocytes and other clotting factors combine. Thrombosis describes the condition of forming a clot.

Suffixes

Suffix	Meaning	Medical Term	Meaning
-al	pertaining to	neural _____	
-algia	pain	arthralgia _____	
-cyte	cell	leukocyte _____	
-ectomy	removal, excision	gastrectomy _____	

-emia	blood condition	leukemia _____ Large numbers of immature, cancerous cells are found in the bloodstream and bone marrow (inner part of bone that makes blood cells).
-gram	record	arthrogram _____ This is an x-ray record of a joint.
-ic	pertaining to	gastric _____
-ism	condition	hyperthyroidism _____ HYPER- means "excessive." The thyroid gland is in the neck. It secretes (makes) a hormone called thyroxine, which helps cells burn food to release energy. See Figure 1–6.
-itis	inflammation	gastroenteritis _____

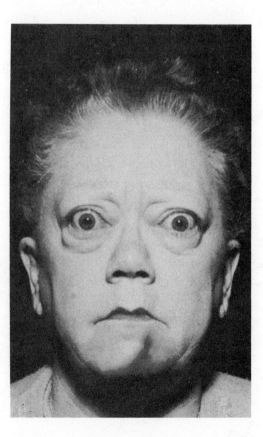

Figure 1–6. Hyperthyroidism: The thyroid gland produces too much hormone and causes symptoms such as rapid pulse, nervousness, excessive sweating, and swelling of tissue behind the eyeball.

-logist	specialist in the study of	neuro<u>logist</u> _____
-logy	study of	nephr<u>ology</u> _____
-oma	tumor, mass	hepat<u>oma</u> _____
-osis	abnormal condition	nephr<u>osis</u> _____
-scope	instrument to visually examine	gastro<u>scope</u> _____
-scopy	process of visual examination	laparo<u>scopy</u> _____ A small incision is made near the navel, and a tube is inserted into the abdomen for viewing organs and doing procedures such as tying off the fallopian tubes. See Figure 1–7. arthro<u>scopy</u> _____ See Figure 1–8.
-sis	state of	progno<u>sis</u> _____
-tomy	process of cutting	neuro<u>tomy</u> _____

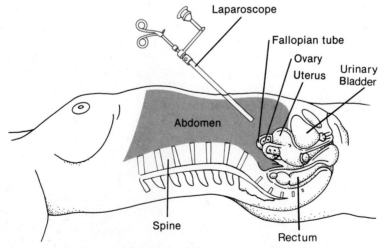

Figure 1–7. Laparoscopy.

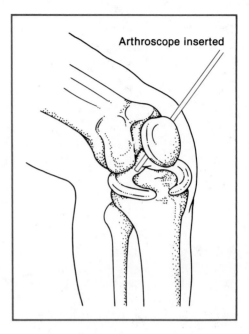

Arthroscope inserted

Figure 1–8. Arthroscopy of the knee.

Prefixes

Prefix	Meaning	Medical Term	Meaning
a-, an-	no, not	anemia	

Literally, *anemia* means a condition of "no blood." Actually, it is a decrease in numbers of red blood cells or a decreased ability to carry oxygen because of less hemoglobin, a protein that helps carry oxygen in red blood cells.

| dia- | complete, through | diagnosis | |

| endo- | within | endocrine glands | |

CRIN/O means "to secrete" (to form and give off). Examples of endocrine glands are the thyroid gland, pituitary gland, adrenal glands, ovaries, and testes. All these glands secrete hormones *into* the bloodstream.

| exo- | outside | exocrine glands | |

Examples of exocrine glands are sweat, tear, and mammary (breast) glands that secrete substances to the *outside* of the body.

hyper-	excessive, more than normal	hyperglycemia _____ GLYC/O means "sugar." Hyperglycemia is also known as diabetes mellitus. *Mellitus* means "sweet."
hypo-	below, less than normal	hypodermic _____ hypoglycemia _____
pro-	before	prognosis _____
re-	back	resection _____ -SECTION means "to cut into an organ" but resection means "to cut an organ out in the sense of cutting back or away." The Latin *resectio* means "a trimming or pruning."
retro-	behind	retrogastric _____
sub-	under, below	subhepatic _____
trans-	across, through	transurethral _____ The urethra is the tube that leads from the urinary bladder to the outside of the body. See Figure 1–2.

III. EXERCISES

These exercises give you practice writing and understanding the terms presented in Section II. An important part of the learning process involves *checking* your answers with the **answer key** given directly after each exercise. The answers are printed close to the questions so that you can easily check your responses. If you can't answer a question, then *please* look at the answer key and *copy* the correct answer. You may want to photocopy some of the exercises before you complete them so that you can practice doing them many times.

A. *Using slashes, divide the following terms into their component parts and give the meaning for the whole term:*

For example: bi/o/logy   study of life

1. adenoma _____

2. arthritis _____

3. enteric _____

4. encephalitis _____

5. dermatosis _____

6. oncologist _____

7. arthroscope _____

8. cerebral _____

9. cardiology _____

10. transhepatic _____

11. cephalic _____

Answer Key: 1. aden/oma — tumor of a gland   2. arthr/itis — inflammation of a joint   3. enter/ic — pertaining to the intestines   4. encephal/itis — inflammation of the brain   5. dermat/osis — abnormal condition of the skin   6. onc/o/logist — specialist in the study of tumors   7. arthr/o/scope — instrument to visually examine a joint   8. cerebr/al — pertaining to the brain or cerebrum, its largest part   9. cardi/o/logy — study of the heart   10. trans/hepat/ic — pertaining to across or through the liver   11. cephal/ic — pertaining to the head

B. *Complete the following medical terms:*

1. _____ gastric   pertaining to under the stomach

2. gastr _____   pain in the stomach

3. gastr _____   inflammation of the stomach

4. _____ gastric   pertaining to across the stomach

5. gastr _____   process of visually examining the stomach

6. _____ gastric   pertaining to behind the stomach

7. gastr _____   instrument to visually examine the stomach

8. gastr _____   study of the stomach and intestines

9. gastr _____   excision (removal) of the stomach

10. gastr _____   incision (to cut into) the stomach

Answer Key: 1. subgastric   2. gastralgia   3. gastritis   4. transgastric
5. gastroscopy   6. retrogastric   7. gastroscope   8. gastroenterology
9. gastrectomy   10. gastrotomy

C. *What part of the body do the following medical terms refer to?*

1. adenoma _____

2. enteritis _____

3. arthrosis _____

4. cerebrovascular accident _____
    (VASCULAR means "pertaining to blood vessels"; a cerebrovascular accident is also
    known as a *stroke,* or *CVA*)

5. dermatitis _____

6. encephalitis _____

7. renal _____

8. osteitis _____

9. nephritis _____

10. electroencephalogram _____

11. rhinitis _____

12. laparotomy _____

13. ophthalmology _____

14. hepatoma _____

D. ***Divide the following terms into component parts and give their meanings:***

1. nephrectomy _____

2. neuritis _____

3. oncology _____

4. gastralgia_____

5. hepatitis_____

6. endocrinology _____
Endocrine glands produce hormones; examples are the thyroid gland in the neck, the pituitary gland at the base of the brain, the ovaries in the female, and the testes in the male.

7. osteoarthritis_____

8. psychology_____

9. dermatosis_____

10. gynecology_____

11. sarcoma_____

12. carcinoma_____

13. transurethral_____

14. ophthalmoscope _____

7. oste/o/arthr/itis — inflammation of bones and joints   8. psych/o/logy — study of the mind   9. dermat/osis — abnormal condition of the skin   10. gynec/o/logy — study of women (disorders of the female reproductive organs)   11. sarc/oma — tumor (cancerous) of flesh tissue   12. carcin/oma — cancerous tumor of skin cells or cells that line the internal organs   13. trans/urethr/al — pertaining to through the urethra (tube that leads from the bladder to the outside of the body) 14. ophthalm/o/scope — instrument to visually examine the eye

E.   Complete the following medical terms:

1. _____ cyte   A **red** blood cell; these cells carry oxygen to all parts of the body.

2. _____ cyte   A **white** blood cell; these cells help to fight disease.

3. _____ cyte   A **clotting** cell; these cells help your blood to clot and are also called *platelets*.

4. _____ gnosis   A state of **complete** knowledge; what your doctor tells you about your condition after testing and examination.

5. _____ thyroidism   A condition of **excessive** production of hormone from the thyroid gland.

6. _____ thyroidism   A condition of **decreased** production of hormone from the thyroid gland.

7. leuk _____   A **blood condition** of too many white blood cells; the cells are cancerous.

8. _____ logy   Study of **nerves** and nervous disorders.

9. _____ oma   Tumor of the **liver.**

10. _____ logy   Study of **disease.**

Answer Key: 1. erythrocyte   2. leukocyte   3. thrombocyte   4. diagnosis   5. hyperthyroidism   6. hypothyroidism   7. leukemia   8. neurology 9. hepatoma   10. pathology

F. *Identify the suffix in each of the following, and give the meaning of the entire term:*

1. osteotomy _____

2. rhinitis _____

3. neuralgia _____

4. nephrosis _____

5. adenectomy _____

6. cerebral _____

7. arthrogram _____

8. laparoscopy _____

9. laparotomy _____

10. hepatitis _____

11. cephalalgia _____

Answer Key: 1. -tomy (process of cutting bone)   2. -itis (inflammation of the nose)   3. -algia (pain of a nerve)   4. -osis (abnormal condition of the kidney)   5. -ectomy (removal of a gland)   6. -al (pertaining to the cerebrum, the largest part of the brain)   7. -gram (record, x-ray, of a joint)   8. -scopy (visual examination of the abdomen)   9. -tomy (incision of the abdomen)   10. -itis (inflammation of the liver)   11. -algia (pain in the head)

G. *Give the meaning for the underlined term in each of the following sentences:*

1. An <u>oncologist</u> treats patients who have sarcomas and carcinomas. _____

    _____

2. After explaining Mr. Green's diagnosis to him and outlining the plan of treatment, Dr.

    Jones' <u>prognosis</u> was hopeful. _____

    _____

3. Seventy-five-year-old Ms. Stein has constant pain in her knees and hips. Her doctor tells her that she has degeneration of her joints and recommends that she take aspirin and and other drugs to reduce discomfort from her <u>osteoarthritis.</u> _____

_____

4. <u>Thrombosis</u> is a serious condition that can lead to blockage of blood vessels. If the blockage stops blood from reaching body cells, those cells die because they are deprived of the food and oxygen that is carried by the blood. _____

_____

5. A <u>pathologist</u> is the medical doctor who specializes in examining biopsy samples and performing autopsies. _____

_____

6. <u>Hyperglycemia</u> can result from a lack of insulin (hormone) secretion from the pancreas (an endocrine gland near the stomach). Without insulin, sugar remains in the blood and cannot enter body cells. _____

_____

7. A patient with a <u>psychosis</u> loses touch with the real world and displays abnormal behavior. _____

_____

8. A doctor uses a cystoscope to perform <u>cystoscopy.</u> _____

_____

9. A <u>laparotomy</u> may be necessary to determine the spread of disease in the abdomen. __

_____

10. The doctor used a <u>laparoscope</u> to cut and tie off Ms. Smith's fallopian tubes so that she couldn't become pregnant. _____

_____

11. Symptoms of <u>hyperthyroidism</u> may include a large thyroid gland and protruding eyeballs (exophthalmia). _____

_____

12. Mr. Paul had a partial <u>resection</u> of his stomach as treatment for his gastric adenocarcinoma. _____

_____

13. <u>Leukemia</u> is diagnosed by looking at a blood sample or taking a bone marrow biopsy.

_____

14. A <u>transurethral</u> resection of the prostate gland is a treatment for overdevelopment of that gland, which is located below the bladder in males. _____

_____

Answer Key: 1. specialist in the study of tumors   2. prediction about the outcome of treatment (literally, "before knowledge")   3. inflammation of bones and joints   4. abnormal condition of clotting or clot formation   5. specialist in the study of disease   6. blood condition of too much sugar   7. abnormal condition of the mind   8. process of visual examination of the urinary bladder   9. incision of the abdomen   10. instrument to visually examine the abdomen   11. condition of too much thyroid hormone   12. removal, excision   13. cancerous condition of white blood cells   14. across (through) the urethra

H. *Circle the term that is spelled correctly and write its meaning:*

1. biospy   biopsy   _____

2. erythrocyte   erithrocyte   _____

3. psychosis   pyschosis   _____

4. ostoarthitis   osteoarthritis _____

5. diagnois   diagnosis   _____

6. platelete   platelet   _____

7.   endocrinology   endocranology   _____

8.   nephroectomy   nephrectomy   _____

9.   nueralgia   neuralgia   _____

10. gastrenterology   gastroenterology   _____

11. opthalmoscope   ophthalmoscope   _____

12. cephalic   cephelic   _____

Answer Key: 1. biopsy — to view life; microscopic examination of living tissue
2. erythrocyte — red blood cell   3. psychosis — abnormal condition of the mind
4. osteoarthritis — inflammation of bones and joints   5. diagnosis — complete
knowledge   6. platelet — clotting cell (thrombocyte)   7. endocrinology — study
of glands that secrete hormones   8. nephrectomy — removal of the kidney
9. neuralgia — pain of a nerve   10. gastroenterology — study of the stomach and
intestines   11. ophthalmoscope — instrument to view the eye   12. cephalic —
pertaining to the head

IV.   REVIEW

Here's your chance to test your understanding of all the **combining forms, suffixes,**
and **prefixes** that you have studied in this chapter. Write the meaning of each term in the
space provided and *check* your answers with the answer key at the end of each list!

COMBINING FORMS

Combining Form	Meaning		Combining Form	Meaning
1. aden/o	_____		6. cephal/o	_____
2. arthr/o	_____		7. cerebr/o	_____
3. bi/o	_____		8. cyst/o	_____
4. carcin/o	_____		9. cyt/o	_____
5. cardi/o	_____		10. dermat/o	_____

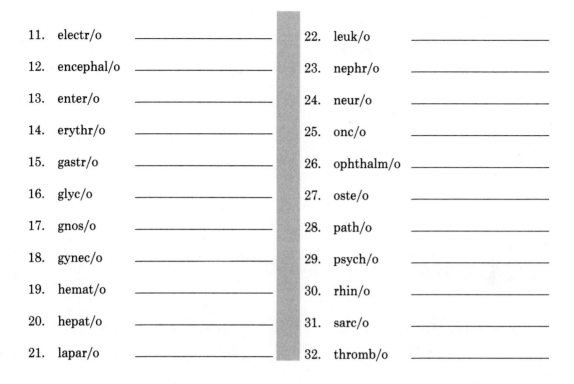

11. electr/o _____

12. encephal/o _____

13. enter/o _____

14. erythr/o _____

15. gastr/o _____

16. glyc/o _____

17. gnos/o _____

18. gynec/o _____

19. hemat/o _____

20. hepat/o _____

21. lapar/o _____

22. leuk/o _____

23. nephr/o _____

24. neur/o _____

25. onc/o _____

26. ophthalm/o _____

27. oste/o _____

28. path/o _____

29. psych/o _____

30. rhin/o _____

31. sarc/o _____

32. thromb/o _____

SUFFIXES

Suffix	*Meaning*		*Suffix*	*Meaning*
1. -al	_____		10. -opsy	_____
2. -algia	_____		11. -ectomy	_____
3. -cyte	_____		12. -emia	_____
4. -ic	_____		13. -scope	_____
5. -ism	_____		14. -scopy	_____
6. -itis	_____		15. -sis	_____
7. -logist	_____		16. -tomy	_____
8. -logy	_____		17. -osis	_____
9. -oma	_____			

PREFIXES

Prefix	Meaning		Prefix	Meaning
1. a-, an-	_____		7. pro-	_____
2. dia-	_____		8. re-	_____
3. endo-	_____		9. retro-	_____
4. exo-	_____		10. sub-	_____
5. hyper-	_____		11. trans-	_____
6. hypo-	_____			

COMBINING FORMS

Answer Key: 1. gland   2. joint   3. life   4. cancerous   5. heart
6. head   7. cerebrum   8. urinary bladder   9. cell   10. skin   11. electricity   12. brain   13. intestines   14. red   15. stomach   16. sugar
17. knowledge   18. woman, female   19. blood   20. liver   21. abdomen   22. white   23. kidney   24. nerve   25. tumor   26. eye
27. bone   28. disease   29. mind   30. nose   31. flesh   32. clot

SUFFIXES

Answer Key: 1. pertaining to   2. pain   3. cell   4. pertaining to   5. condition   6. inflammation   7. specialist in the study of   8. study of
9. tumor, mass   10. process of viewing   11. removal   12. blood condition
13. instrument to visually examine   14. process of visual examination
15. condition   16. incision, to cut into   17. abnormal condition

PREFIXES

Answer Key: 1. no, not   2. complete   3. within   4. out, outside   5. too
much, above   6. below, too little, deficient   7. before   8. back   9. behind   10. under, below   11. across, through

V. PRONUNCIATION OF TERMS

The terms that you have learned in this chapter are presented here with their pronunciations. The capitalized letters in boldface are the accented syllable. Write the meaning of each term next to its pronunciation.

Term	Pronunciation	Meaning
adenitis	ad-eh-**NI**-tis	
adenoma	ah-deh-**NO**-mah	
anemia	ah-**NE**-me-ah	
arthralgia	ar-**THRAL**-je-ah	
arthritis	ar-**THRI**-tis	
arthrogram	**AR**-thro-gram	
arthroscope	**AR**-thro-skop	
arthroscopy	ar-**THROS**-ko-pe	
biology	bi-**OL**-o-je	
biopsy	**BI**-op-se	
carcinoma	kar-sih-**NO**-mah	
cardiac	**KAR**-de-ak	
cardiology	kar-de-**OL**-o-je	
cephalic	seh-**FAL**-ik	
cerebral	seh-**RE**-bral	
cerebrovascular accident	seh-re-bro-**VAS**-ku-lar **AK**-sih-dent	
cystoscope	**SIS**-to-skop	
cystoscopy	sis-**TOS**-ko-pe	
cytology	sī-**TOL**-o-je	

dermatitis	der-mah-**TI**-tis	_____
dermatosis	der-mah-**TO**-sis	_____
diagnosis	di-ag-**NO**-sis	_____
electrocardiogram	e-lek-tro-**KAR**-de-o-gram	_____
electroencephalogram	e-lek-tro-en-**SEF**-ah-lo-gram	_____
endocrine glands	**EN**-do-krin glanz	_____
enteritis	en-ter-**I**-tis	_____
erythrocyte	eh-**RITH**-ro-sīt	_____
exocrine glands	**EK**-so-krin glanz	_____
gastrectomy	gas-**TREK**-to-me	_____
gastric	**GAS**-trik	_____
gastritis	gas-**TRI**-tis	_____
gastroenteritis	gas-tro-en-teh-**RI**-tis	_____
gastroenterology	gas-tro-en-ter-**OL**-o-je	_____
gastroscope	**GAS**-tro-skop	_____
gastroscopy	gas-**TROS**-ko-pe	_____
gastrotomy	gas-**TROT**-o-me	_____
gynecologist	gi-neh-**KOL**-o-jist	_____
gynecology	gi-neh-**KOL**-o-je	_____
hematoma	he-mah-**TO**-mah	_____
hepatitis	hep-ah-**TI**-tis	_____
hepatoma	hep-ah-**TO**-mah	_____
hyperglycemia	hi-per-gli-**SE**-me-ah	_____

hyperthyroidism	hi-per-**THI**-royd-izm _____
hypodermic	hi-po-**DER**-mik _____
hypoglycemia	hi-po-gli-**SE**-me-ah _____
hypothyroidism	hi-po-**THI**-royd-izm _____
laparoscopy	lap-ah-**ROS**-ko-pe _____
laparotomy	lap-ah-**ROT**-o-me _____
leukemia	lu-**KE**-me-ah _____
leukocyte	**LU**-ko-sīt _____
nephrectomy	neh-**FREK**-to-me _____
nephrology	neh-**FROL**-o-je _____
nephrosis	neh-**FRO**-sis _____
neural	**NU**-ral _____
neuralgia	nu-**RAL**-je-ah _____
neuritis	nu-**RI**-tis _____
neurology	nur-**ROL**-o-je _____
neurotomy	nur-**ROT**-o-me _____
oncologist	ong-**KOL**-o-jist _____
ophthalmoscope	of-**THAL**-mo-skop _____
osteitis	os-te-**I**-tis _____
osteoarthritis	os-te-o-ar-**THRI**-tis _____
pathologist	pah-**THOL**-o-jist _____
platelet	**PLAT**-let _____
prognosis	prog-**NO**-sis _____

psychosis	sī-**KO**-sis _____
renal	**RE**-nal _____
resection	re-**SEK**-shun _____
retrogastric	reh-tro-**GAS**-trik _____
rhinitis	ri-**NI**-tis _____
rhinotomy	ri-**NOT**-o-me _____
sarcoma	sar-**KO**-mah _____
subgastric	sub-**GAS**-trik _____
subhepatic	sub-heh-**PAT**-ik _____
thrombocyte	**THROM**-bo-sīt _____
thrombosis	throm-**BO**-sis _____
transgastric	trans-**GAS**-trik _____
transurethral	trans-u-**RE**-thral _____

CHAPTER 2

ORGANIZATION OF THE BODY

CHAPTER OBJECTIVES

- To name the body systems and their functions
- To identify body cavities and specific organs within them
- To list the divisions of the back
- To identify three planes of the body
- To analyze, pronounce, and spell new terms related to organs and tissues in the body

---

I. BODY SYSTEMS

All parts of your body are composed of individual units called **cells.** Muscle, nerve, skin (epithelial), and bone cells are some examples.

Similar cells grouped together are **tissues.** Groups of muscle cells are muscle tissue, and groups of epithelial cells are epithelial tissue.

Collections of different tissues working together are called **organs.** An organ, such as the stomach, has different tissues (muscle, epithelial, nerve tissues) that help the organ function.

Groups of organs working together are the **systems** of the body. The digestive system, for example, includes organs such as the mouth, throat, esophagus, stomach, and intestines which bring food into the body and deliver it to the bloodstream.

There are ten systems of the body, and each plays an important role in the way the body works.

The **circulatory system** (the heart, blood, and blood vessels such as arteries, veins, and capillaries) transports blood throughout the body. The circulatory system also includes lymph vessels and nodes that carry a clear fluid called lymph. Lymph contains white blood cells called lymphocytes that fight against disease.

The **digestive system** brings food into the body and breaks it down so that it can enter the bloodstream. Food that cannot be broken down is then removed from the body at the end of the system.

The **endocrine system,** made up of glands, sends chemical messengers, called hormones, into the blood to act on other glands and organs.

The **female and male reproductive systems** produce the cells that join to form the beginning of a new baby.

The **musculoskeletal system,** including muscles, bones, joints, and connective tissues, supports the body and allows it to move.

The **nervous system** carries electrical messages to and from the brain and spinal cord.

The **respiratory system** controls breathing, which allows air to enter and leave the body.

The **skin and sense organ system,** including the skin and eyes and ears, receives messages from the environment and sends them to the brain.

The **urinary system** produces urine and sends it out of the body through the kidneys, bladder, and other tubes.

Appendix I, at the back of the book, contains diagrams of each body system. The *Glossary of Medical Terms* contains the definitions of organs pictured in the diagrams, and the *Glossary of Word Parts* gives combining forms used to describe the organs. Use the appendix and glossaries as references during your study and later when you work in the medical field.

II. BODY CAVITIES

Figure 2–1 shows the five body cavities. A body cavity is a space containing organs. Label Figure 2–1 as you read the following paragraphs.

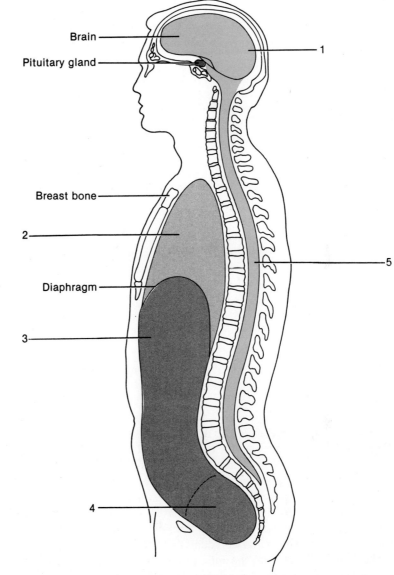

Brain

Pituitary gland

1

Breast bone

2

Diaphragm

3

5

4

Figure 2–1. Body cavities.

The **cranial cavity** (1) is located in the head and is surrounded by the skull (CRANI/O means "skull"). The brain and other organs, such as the pituitary gland (an endocrine gland below the brain), are in the cranial cavity.

The **thoracic cavity** (2) is the chest cavity (THORAC/O means "chest"), which is surrounded by the breast bone and ribs. The lungs, heart, windpipe (trachea), bronchial tubes (leading from the trachea to the lungs), and other organs are in the thoracic cavity.

Figure 2–2 shows a front view of the thoracic cavity. The lungs are each surrounded by a double membrane called the **pleura.** The space between the pleura and surrounding each

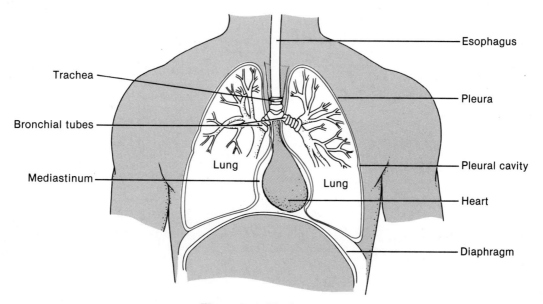

Figure 2–2. Thoracic cavity.

lung is called the **pleural cavity.** The large space between the lungs is called the **mediastinum.** The heart, esophagus (food tube), trachea, and bronchial tubes are organs within the mediastinum.

Returning to Figure 2–1, the **abdominal cavity** (3) is the space below the thoracic cavity. The **diaphragm** is the muscle that separates the abdominal and thoracic cavities. Organs in the abdomen include the stomach, liver, gallbladder, and small and large intestines.

The organs in the abdomen are covered by a membrane called the **peritoneum** (see Figure 2–3). The peritoneum attaches the abdominal organs to the abdominal muscles and surrounds each organ to hold it in place.

Turn back to Figure 2–1 and locate the **pelvic cavity** (4), below the abdominal cavity. The pelvic cavity is surrounded by the **pelvis** (hip bone). Organs that are located within the pelvic cavity are the urinary bladder, ureters (tubes from the kidneys to the bladder), urethra (tube from the bladder to the outside of the body), rectum and anus, and the uterus (muscular organ that nourishes the developing fetus) in females.

Figure 2–1 also shows the **spinal cavity** (5). This is the space surrounded by the **spinal column** (backbones). The **spinal cord** is the nervous tissue within the spinal cavity. Nerves enter and leave the spinal cord carrying messages to and from all parts of the body.

As a quick review of the terms presented in this section, write the term from the list next to its meaning on the space provided.

Term		*Meaning*
Abdominal cavity	1.	Membrane surrounding the lungs _____
Cranial cavity	2.	Space between the lungs, containing the heart _____

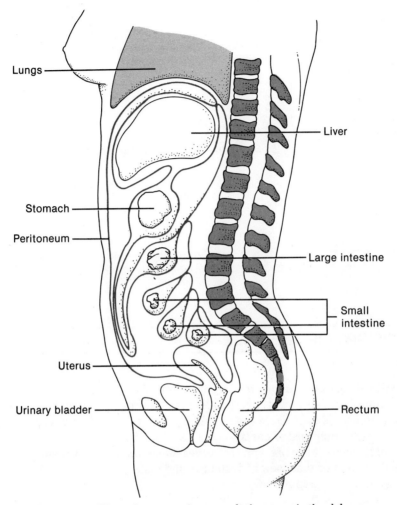

Figure 2–3. The peritoneum as it surrounds the organs in the abdomen.

Diaphragm
Mediastinum
Pelvic cavity
Pelvis
Peritoneum
Pleura
Spinal cavity
Thoracic cavity

3. Hip bone _____

4. Space containing the liver, gallbladder, and stomach; also called the abdomen _____

5. Space within the backbones, containing the spinal cord _____

6. Membrane surrounding the organs in the abdomen _____

7. Space within the skull, containing the brain _____

8. Space below the abdominal cavity, containing the urinary bladder _____

9. Muscle between the thoracic and abdominal cavities _____

10. Entire chest cavity, containing the lungs, heart, trachea, esophagus, and bronchial tubes _____

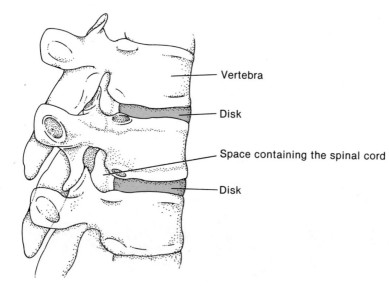

— Vertebra

— Disk

— Space containing the spinal cord

— Disk

Figure 2–4. Vertebrae and disks.

III. DIVISIONS OF THE BACK

The **spinal column** is a long row of bones from the neck to the tailbone. Each bone in the spinal column is called a **vertebra** (backbone). Two or more bones are **vertebrae.**

A piece of flexible connective tissue, called a **disk** (also spelled disc), lies between each backbone. The disk, composed of **cartilage,** is a cushion between the bones. If the disk slips, or moves out of its place, it can press on the nerves that enter or leave the spinal cord and cause pain. Figure 2–4 shows a side view of vertebrae and disks.

The divisions of the spinal column are pictured in Figure 2–5. Label them according to the following list:

Division	*Bones*	*Abbreviation*
1. **Cervical** (neck) region	7 bones	C1–C7
2. **Thoracic** (chest) region	12 bones	T1–T12
3. **Lumbar** (loin or waist) region	5 bones	L1–L5
4. **Sacral** (sacrum or lower back) region	5 fused bones	S1–S5
5. **Coccygeal** (coccyx or tailbone) region	4 fused bones	

IV. PLANES OF THE BODY

A plane is an imaginary flat surface. Organs appear in different relationships to each other according to the plane of the body in which they are viewed.

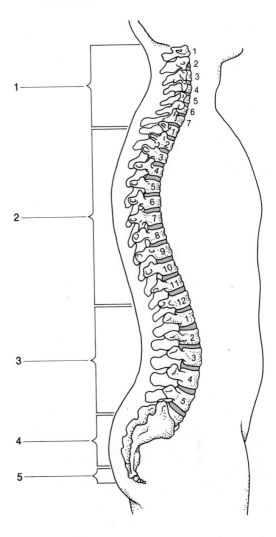

Figure 2–5. The divisions of the back.

Figure 2–6 shows three planes of the body. Label them as you read the following descriptions:

1. **Frontal plane** (sometimes called the coronal plane) — An up-and-down plane that divides the body or organ into front **(anterior)** and back **(posterior)** portions. A routine chest x-ray shows the thoracic cavity in the frontal plane. Figure 2–2 shows organs in the frontal plane.

2. **Sagittal plane** — A plane that divides the body or an organ into a right and left side. Figures 2–1, 2–3, and 2–5 show the body in a sagittal plane, or **lateral** (side) view.

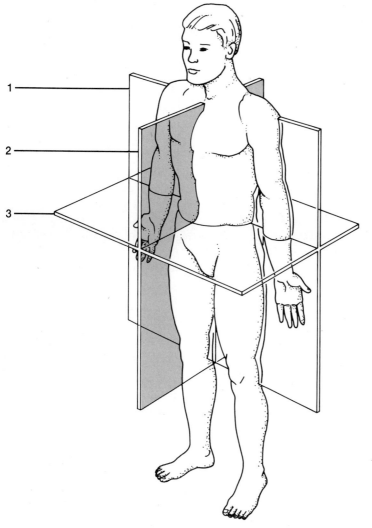

Figure 2–6. Planes of the body.

3. **Transverse plane**   A plane that divides the body or organ into upper and lower portions, as in a **cross-section. A CT scan** (CAT scan) is an x-ray picture of the body taken in the transverse plane. Figure 2–7 is a CT scan of the brain.

    Magnetic resonance imaging (MRI) is the latest technique of producing images of the body. No x-rays are used, but pictures are made by using magnetic waves. The images from MRI show organs in all three planes (frontal, sagittal, and transverse) of the body (see Figure 2–8).

Figure 2 – 7. CT scan of the brain. Notice the large white region in the brain indicating an area of dead tissue, where a stroke (cerebrovascular accident) has occurred. The figure of the man with the line across his head shows you the transverse plane of the CT scan.

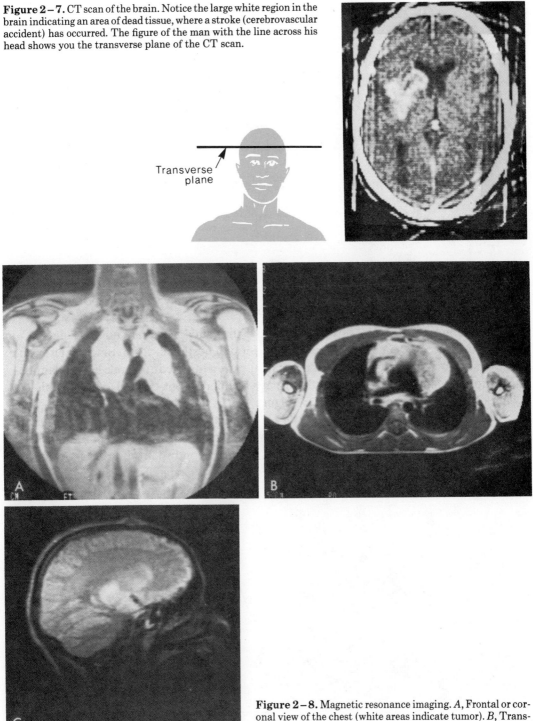

Transverse plane

Figure 2 – 8. Magnetic resonance imaging. *A*, Frontal or coronal view of the chest (white areas indicate tumor). *B*, Transverse view of the chest. *C*, Sagittal (lateral) view of the brain.

V.   TERMINOLOGY

Write the meanings of the medical terms on the line provided. Check the meanings with the *Glossary* at the end of the book or with a medical dictionary.

Combining Form	Meaning	Medical Term	Meaning
abdomin/o	abdomen	abdominal _____	
bronch/o	bronchial tubes (lead from the windpipe to the lungs)	bronchoscopy _____	
cervic/o	*neck* of the body or *neck* (cervix) of the uterus	cervical _____	

cervical _____
You must decide from the context of what you are reading whether *cervical* means "pertaining to the neck of the body" or "pertaining to the cervix" (lower portion of the uterus). Figure 2–9 shows the uterus and the cervix.

coccyg/o	coccyx, tailbone	coccygeal _____	
crani/o	skull	craniotomy _____	

coccygeal _____
-EAL means "pertaining to."

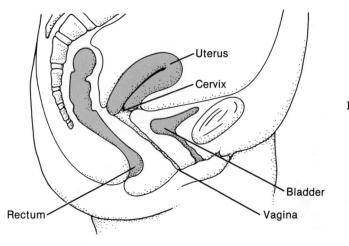

Figure 2–9. The uterus and cervix.

Uterus
Cervix
Bladder
Rectum
Vagina

epitheli/o	skin, surface tissue	epithelial _____ The term *epithelial* was first used to describe the surface (*epi* means "upon") of the breast nipple (*thele* means "nipple"). Now it is used to describe all body surfaces and linings of internal organs that lead to the outside of the body.
esophag/o	esophagus (tube from the throat to the stomach)	esophageal _____
hepat/o	liver	hepatitis _____
lapar/o	abdomen	laparoscopy _____ laparotomy _____
laryng/o	larynx (voice box)	laryngeal _____ The larynx (**LAR**-inks) is found in the upper part of the trachea. laryngectomy _____
later/o	side	lateral _____
lumb/o	loin (waist)	lumbar _____ -AR means "pertaining to." A lumbar puncture is the placement of a needle within the membranes in the lumbar region of the spinal cord to withdraw fluid.
lymph/o	lymph (clear fluid in tissue spaces and lymph vessels)	lymphocyte _____ Lymphocytes are white blood cells and are important in fighting disease.
mediastin/o	mediastinum (space between the lungs)	mediastinal _____
pelv/o	pelvis (hip bone)	pelvic _____

peritone/o	peritoneum (membrane surrounding the abdomen)	peritoneal _____
pharyng/o	pharynx (throat)	pharyngeal _____ The pharynx (**FAR**-inks) is the common passageway for food from the mouth and air from the nose.
pleur/o	pleura	pleuritis _____
sacr/o	sacrum (five fused bones in the lower back)	sacral _____
spin/o	spine (backbone)	spinal _____
thorac/o	chest	thoracotomy _____ thoracic _____
trache/o	trachea (windpipe)	tracheotomy _____
vertebr/o	vertebra (backbone)	vertebral _____

VI.   EXERCISES

A.   Match the following systems of the body with their functions:

digestive   musculoskeletal   circulatory
respiratory   urinary   endocrine
skin and sense organs   nervous   reproductive

1.   Produces urine and sends it out of the body: _____

2.   Secretes hormones that are carried by blood to other organs: _____

3.   Supports the body and helps it move: _____

4. Takes food into the body and breaks it down: _____

5. Transports food, gases, and other substances through the body: _____

_____

6. Moves air in and out of the body: _____

7. Produces the cells that unite to form a new baby: _____

8. Receives messages from the environment and sends them to the brain: _____

_____

9. Carries electrical messages to and from the brain and spinal cord: _____

_____

Answer Key: 1. urinary   2. endocrine   3. musculoskeletal   4. digestive
5. circulatory   6. respiratory   7. reproductive   8. skin and sense organs
9. nervous

B. *Use the following terms to complete the chart below. Give the name of the*
cavity and an organ that is contained within the cavity.

spinal cavity	pelvic cavity	cranial cavity
thoracic cavity	abdominal cavity	urinary bladder
stomach	lungs	spinal cord
brain	uterus	heart

	Cavity	*Organ*
1. Space contained within the hip bone	_____	_____
2. Space contained within the skull	_____	_____
3. Space contained within the chest	_____	_____
4. Space contained within the abdomen	_____	_____
5. Space contained within the backbones	_____	_____

C.   *Complete the following sentences using the terms listed below.*

mediastinum	pelvis	vertebra
diaphragm	spinal cord	spinal column
disk	peritoneum	abdomen (abdominal cavity)
		pleura

1.   The hip bone is the _____.

2.   The muscle separating the chest and the abdomen is the _____.

3.   The membrane surrounding the organs in the abdomen is the _____.

4.   The membrane surrounding the lungs is the _____.

5.   The space between the lungs in the chest is the _____.

6.   The space that contains organs such as the stomach, liver, gallbladder, and intestines is

the _____.

7.   The backbones are called the _____.

8.   The nerves running down the back are called the _____.

9.   A single backbone is called a _____.

10.   A piece of cartilage in between each backbone is called a _____.

D. Name the five divisions of the spinal column from the neck to the tailbone:

1. C _ _ _ _ _ _ _

2. T _ _ _ _ _ _ _

3. L _ _ _ _ _

4. S _ _ _ _ _

5. C _ _ _ _ _ _ _

Answer Key: 1. Cervical   2. Thoracic   3. Lumbar   4. Sacral   5. Coccy-geal

E. Match the following terms with their meanings below.

transverse plane   CT scan   anterior
frontal plane   sagittal plane   posterior
MRI   cartilage   lateral

1. Pertaining to the back: _____

2. Pertaining to the front: _____

3. A plane that divides the body into an upper and lower part: _____

4. Pertaining to the side: _____

5. A picture of the body using magnetic waves; all three planes of the body can be viewed:

    _____

6. A plane that divides the body into right and left parts: _____

7. Flexible connective tissue found between bones at joints: _____

8. A plane that divides the body into front and back parts: _____

9. Series of x-ray pictures taken in cross-section: _____

F. **Give meanings for the following medical terms:**

1. craniotomy _____

2. abdominal _____

3. pelvic _____

4. thoracic _____

5. mediastinal _____

6. epithelial _____

7. tracheotomy _____

8. peritoneal _____

9. hepatitis _____

10. cervical _____

11. lymphocyte _____

12. lateral _____

13. bronchoscopy _____

G. Select from the following to complete the sentences below:

pleuritis	pharyngeal	laryngeal	esophageal
epithelial	coccygeal	thoracotomy	lumbar
vertebral	laparoscopy	laparotomy	sacral

1. Pertaining to the loin (waist) region directly under the thoracic vertebrae: _____

   _____

2. Pertaining to skin or surface cells: _____

3. Incision of the abdomen: _____

4. Pertaining to the food tube: _____

5. Pertaining to the voice box: _____

6. Inflammation of the membrane surrounding the lungs: _____

7. Pertaining to the throat: _____

8. Pertaining to the sacrum: _____

9. Incision of the chest: _____

10. Pertaining to the tailbone: _____

11. Visual examination of the abdomen: _____

12. Pertaining to backbones: _____

Answer Key: 1. lumbar   2. epithelial   3. laparotomy   4. esophageal
5. laryngeal   6. pleuritis   7. pharyngeal   8. sacral   9. thoracotomy
10. coccygeal   11. laparoscopy   12. vertebral

H. Circle the term that is spelled correctly and give its meaning on the line provided.

1. ploura   pleura   _____

2. peritoneum   peritonum   _____

3. servical   cervical   _____

4. abdomine   abdomen   _____

5. diaphagm   diaphragm   _____

6. lumbar   lumber   _____

7. cartiledge   cartilage   _____

8. thoracic   thorasic   _____

9. larnyx   larynx   _____

10. pharyngeal   pharingeal   _____

11. uterous   uterus   _____

12. ovaries   overies   _____

13. bronchial tubes broncheal tubes _____

14. crainotomy   craniotomy   _____

15. lymphocyte   limphocyte   _____

Answer Key: 1. pleura — the membrane surrounding the lungs   2. peritoneum — the membrane surrounding the organs in the abdominal cavity   3. cervical — pertaining to the neck of the body, or the neck of the uterus (cervix)   4. abdomen — space below the chest containing organs such as the stomach, intestines, liver, gallbladder, and spleen   5. diaphragm — muscle separating the abdomen from the chest.   6. lumbar — pertaining to the loin (waist) region of the back   7. cartilage — flexible, connective tissue at joints   8. thoracic — pertaining to the chest 9. larynx — voice box   10. pharyngeal — pertaining to the throat   11. uterus — womb   12. ovaries — glands that produce egg cells and hormones   13. bronchial tubes — tubes that carry air from the windpipe to the lungs   14. craniotomy — incision of the skull   15. lymphocyte — lymph cell

VII. REVIEW

Write the meanings of the following combining forms and suffixes. Be sure to check your answers.

COMBINING FORMS

Combining Form	Meaning	Combining Form	Meaning
1. abdomin/o	_____	13. lymph/o	_____
2. bronch/o	_____	14. mediastin/o	_____
3. cervic/o	_____	15. pelv/o	_____
4. coccyg/o	_____	16. peritone/o	_____
5. crani/o	_____	17. pharyng/o	_____
6. epitheli/o	_____	18. pleur/o	_____
7. esophag/o	_____	19. sacr/o	_____
8. hepat/o	_____	20. spin/o	_____
9. lapar/o	_____	21. thorac/o	_____
10. laryng/o	_____	22. trache/o	_____
11. later/o	_____	23. vertebr/o	_____
12. lumb/o	_____		

SUFFIXES

Suffix	Meaning	Suffix	Meaning
1. -ac	_____	4. -cyte	_____
2. -al	_____	5. -eal	_____
3. -ar	_____	6. -ectomy	_____

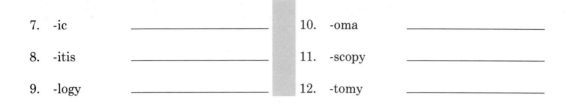

7. -ic _____   10. -oma _____

8. -itis _____   11. -scopy _____

9. -logy _____   12. -tomy _____

COMBINING FORMS

Answer Key: 1. abdomen   2. bronchial tubes   3. neck   4. tailbone
5. skull   6. skin   7. esophagus   8. liver   9. abdomen   10. voice
box   11. side   12. loin, waist region   13. lymph   14. mediastinum
15. hip bone   16. peritoneum   17. throat   18. pleura   19. sacrum
20. backbone   21. chest   22. windpipe   23. backbone

SUFFIXES

Answer Key: 1. pertaining to   2. pertaining to   3. pertaining to   4. cell
5. pertaining to   6. removal, excision, resection   7. pertaining to   8. inflammation   9. study of   10. tumor, mass   11. process of viewing   12. incision, to cut into

VIII. PRONUNCIATION OF TERMS

Write the meaning of each term on the line provided.

abdomen	**AB**-do-men _____
abdominal cavity	ab-**DOM**-in-al **KAV**-i-te_____
anterior	an-**TE**-re-or _____
bronchial tubes	**BRONG**-ke-al tubes _____

bronchoscopy	bron-**KOS**-ko-pe _____
cartilage	**KAR**-ti-lij _____
cervical	**SER**-vi-kal _____
circulatory system	**SER**-ku-lah-tor-e **SIS**-tem _____
coccygeal	kok-sih-**JE**-al _____
coccyx	**KOK**-siks _____
cranial cavity	**KRA**-ne-al **KAV**-ih-te _____
craniotomy	kra-ne-**OT**-o-me _____
diaphragm	**DI**-ah-fram _____
digestive system	di-**JES**-tiv **SIS**-tem _____
disk (disc)	disk _____
endocrine system	**EN**-do-krin **SIS**-tem _____
epithelial	ep-ih-**THE**-le-al _____
esophageal	eh-sof-ah-**JE**-al _____
esophagus	eh-**SOF**-ah-gus _____
female reproductive system	**FE**-mal re-pro-**DUK**-tive **SIS**-tem _____
frontal section	**FRON**-tal **SEK**-shun _____
hepatitis	hep-ah-**TI**-tis _____
laparoscopy	lap-ah-**ROS**-ko-pe _____
laparotomy	lap-ah-**ROT**-o-me _____
laryngeal	lah-rin-**JE**-al _____
laryngectomy	lah-rin-**JEK**-to-me _____

larynx	**LAR**-inks
lateral	**LAT**-er-al
lumbar	**LUM**-bar
lymphocyte	**LIMF**-o-sīt
mediastinal	me-de-ah-**STI**-nal
mediastinum	me-de-ah-**STI**-num
musculoskeletal system	mus-ku-lo-**SKEL**-e-tal **SIS**-tem
nervous system	**NER**-vus **SIS**-tem
ovary	**O**-vah-re
pelvic cavity	**PEL**-vik **KAV**-ih-te
pelvis	**PEL**-vis
peritoneal	per-ih-to-**NE**-al
peritoneum	per-ih-to-**NE**-um
pharyngeal	fah-rin-**JE**-al
pharynx	**FAR**-inks
pituitary gland	pih-**TU**-ih-tah-re gland
pleura	**PLOOR**-ah
pleuritis	ploo-**RI**-tis
posterior	pos-**TER**-e-or
respiratory system	**RES**-pir-ah-tor-e **SIS**-tem
sacral	**SA**-kral
sacrum	**SA**-krum
sagittal plane	**SAJ**-ih-tal plan

spinal cavity	**SPI**-nal **KAV**-ih-te _____
spinal column	**SPI**-nal **KOL**-um _____
spinal cord	**SPI**-nal kord _____
thoracic cavity	tho-**RAS**-ik **KAV**-ih-te _____
thoracotomy	tho-rah-**KOT**-o-me _____
trachea	**TRAY**-ke-ah _____
tracheotomy	tray-ke-**OT**-o-me _____
ureter	**U**-reh-ter _____
urethra	u-**RE**-thrah _____
urinary system	**UR**-in-er-e **SIS**-tem _____
uterus	**U**-ter-us _____
vertebra	**VER**-teh-brah _____
vertebrae	**VER**-teh-bray _____
vertebral	**VER**-teh-bral _____

CHAPTER 3

SUFFIXES

CHAPTER OBJECTIVES

- To identify and define useful diagnostic and procedural suffixes
- To analyze, spell, and pronounce medical terms that contain diagnostic and procedural suffixes

I. INTRODUCTION

This chapter reviews the suffixes that you have learned in the first two chapters and also introduces new suffixes and medical terms. The combining forms used in the chapter are listed below in Section II. Check the list and underline the combining forms that are completely new to you. Refer to this list as you write the meanings of the terms in Section III. Be faithful about completing the exercises in Section IV, and remember to check your answers! These exercises will help you spell terms correctly and understand their meanings. Test yourself by completing the review in Section V and Pronunciation of Terms in Section VI.

II. COMBINING FORMS

Combining Form	Meaning
aden/o	gland
amni/o	amnion (sac of fluid surrounding the embryo)
angi/o	vessel (usually a blood vessel)
arteri/o	artery
arthr/o	joint
ather/o	plaque (a yellow, fatty material)
axill/o	armpit (underarm)
bronch/o	bronchial tubes
bronchi/o	bronchial tubes
carcin/o	cancerous
cardi/o	heart
chem/o	drug (or chemical)
cholecyst/o	gallbladder
chron/o	time
col/o	colon (large intestine or bowel)
crani/o	skull
cyst/o	urinary bladder; also a sac of fluid or cyst
electr/o	electricity
encephal/o	brain
erythr/o	red
esophag/o	esophagus (tube leading from the throat to the stomach)
hem/o	blood
hemat/o	blood
hepat/o	liver
hyster/o	uterus
inguin/o	groin (the depression between the thigh and the trunk of the body)
isch/o	to hold back
lapar/o	abdomen (abdominal wall)
laryng/o	voice box (larynx)

leuk/o	white
mamm/o	breast (use with -ary, -graphy, -gram, and -plasty)
mast/o	breast (use with -ectomy and -itis)
men/o	menses (menstruation); month
mening/o	meninges (membranes around the brain and spinal cord)
my/o	muscle
myel/o	spinal cord (nervous tissue connected to the brain and located within the spinal column or backbone); in some terms, myel/o means bone marrow (the soft, inner part of bones, where blood cells are made)
necr/o	death (of cells)
nephr/o	kidney (use with all suffixes, except -al and -gram; use ren/o with -al and -gram)
neur/o	nerve
oophor/o	ovary
oste/o	bone
ot/o	ear
pelv/o	pelvic bone (hip bone)
peritone/o	peritoneum (membrane surrounding the organs in the abdominal cavity)
pneumon/o	lung
radi/o	x-rays
ren/o	kidney (use with -al and -gram)
rhin/o	nose
salping/o	fallopian (uterine) tubes
sarc/o	flesh
septic/o	pertaining to infection
thorac/o	chest
tonsill/o	tonsils
trache/o	windpipe; trachea
ur/o	urine or urea (waste material); urinary tract
vascul/o	blood vessel

III.   SUFFIXES AND TERMINOLOGY

Suffixes are divided into two groups, those that describe **diagnoses** and those that describe **procedures.**

Diagnostic Suffixes

These suffixes describe disease conditions or their symptoms. Use the list of combining forms in the previous section to write the meaning of each term. You will find it helpful to check the meanings of the terms with the *glossary* at the end of book or with a medical dictionary.

Noun Suffix	Meaning	Terminology	Meaning
-algia	pain	arthralgia _____	
		otalgia _____	
		myalgia _____	
		neuralgia _____	
-emia	blood condition	leukemia _____ Increase in numbers of leukocytes; cells are malignant (cancerous).	
		septicemia _____	
		ischemia _____ Figure 3–1 illustrates ischemia of heart muscle caused by blockage of a coronary (heart) artery.	

Coronary artery occlusion ——

Area of ischemia ——

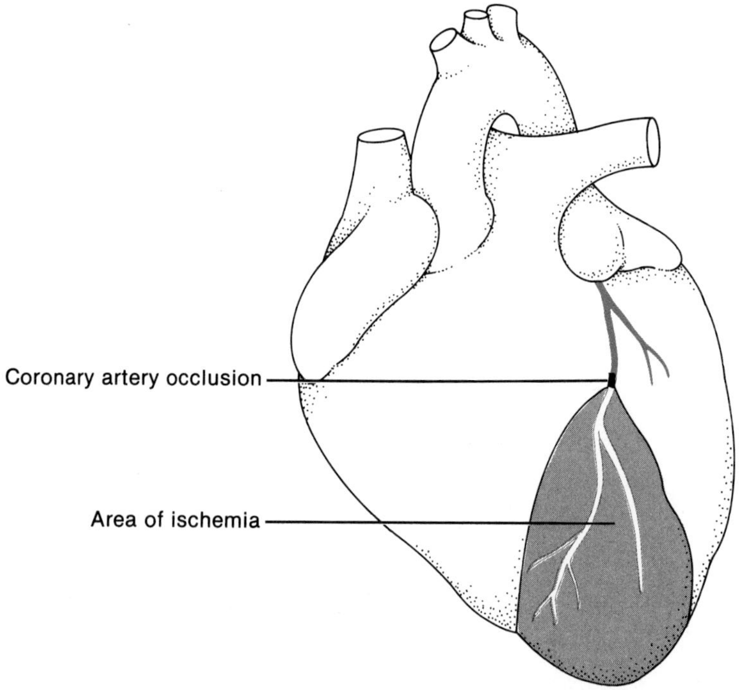

Figure 3–1. Ischemia of heart muscle. Blood is held back from an area of heart muscle by an occlusion (blockage) of a coronary (heart) artery. The muscle then loses its supply of oxygen and food and, if the condition persists, dies. The death of the heart muscle is known as a heart attack (myocardial infarction).

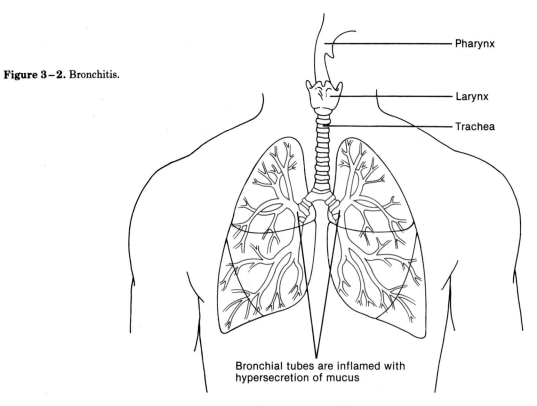

Figure 3–2. Bronchitis.

Pharynx

Larynx

Trachea

Bronchial tubes are inflamed with hypersecretion of mucus

		uremia _____ Uremia occurs when the kidneys fail to function.
-ia	condition, disease	pneumonia _____
-itis	inflammation	bronchitis _____ See Figure 3–2.
		esophagitis _____
		laryngitis _____
		meningitis _____ The meninges are membranes that surround and protect the brain and spinal cord. See Figure 3–3.
		cystitis _____

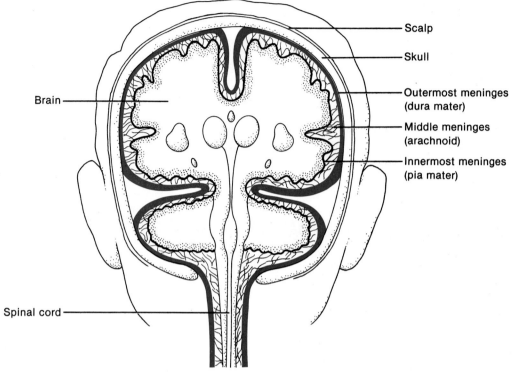

Figure 3–3. Meninges (frontal view).

Noun Suffix	Meaning	Terminology	Meaning
		colitis _____	
		Table 3–1 lists other common inflammatory conditions with their meanings.	
-megaly	enlargement	cardiomegaly _____	
		hepatomegaly _____	
-osis	condition, abnormal condition	nephrosis _____	
		necrosis _____	
		erythrocytosis _____	
		When -OSIS is used with blood cell words it means "a slight increase in numbers of cells."	

Table 3-1. Inflammations

appendicitis	Inflammation of the appendix (hangs from the colon in the lower right abdomen)
bursitis	Inflammation of a small sac of fluid (bursa) near a joint
cellulitis	Inflammation of soft tissue
endocarditis	Inflammation of the inner lining of the heart (endocardium)
epiglottitis	Inflammation of the epiglottis (cartilage at the upper part of the windpipe)
gastritis	Inflammation of the stomach
hepatitis	Inflammation of the liver
myositis	Inflammation of muscle
nephritis	Inflammation of the kidney
osteomyelitis	Inflammation of bone and bone marrow
otitis	Inflammation of the ear
pharyngitis	Inflammation of the throat
thrombophlebitis	Inflammation of a vein with formation of clots

-oma	tumor, mass	adenoma _____

adenoma _____
This is a benign (non-cancerous) tumor

adenocarcinoma _____
Carcinomas are malignant (cancerous) tumors of epithelial (skin) tissue in the body. Glands and the linings of internal organs are composed of epithelial tissue.

myoma _____
This is a benign tumor.

myosarcoma _____
Sarcomas are cancerous tumors of connective (flesh) tissue. Muscle, bone, cartilage, and fat are examples of connective tissues.

hematoma _____
This is not a tumor but a collection of fluid (blood).

-pathy   disease

encephalopathy _____
Pronunciation is en-sef-ah-**LOP**-ah-the.

cardiomyopathy _____
Pronunciation is kar-de-o-mi-**OP**-ah-the.

nephropathy _____
Pronunciation is neh-**FROP**-ah-the.

-rrhea	flow, discharge	rhino<u>rrhea</u> _____
		meno<u>rrhea</u> _____ Normal menstrual flow.
-rrhage or -rrhagia	bursting forth of blood	hemo<u>rrhage</u> _____
		meno<u>rrhagia</u> _____ Excessive bleeding during menstruation.
-sclerosis	hardening	arterio<u>sclerosis</u> _____ *Atherosclerosis* is the most common type of arteriosclerosis. A fatty plaque collects on the lining of arteries. See Figure 3–4.
-uria	condition of urine	hemat<u>uria</u> _____ Bleeding into the urinary tract can cause this condition.

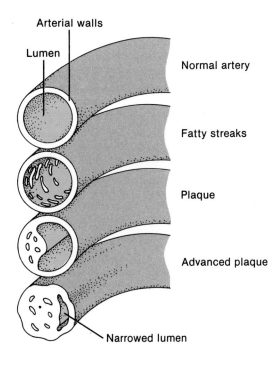

Arterial walls

Lumen

Normal artery

Fatty streaks

Plaque

Advanced plaque

Narrowed lumen

Figure 3–4. Atherosclerosis (type of arteriosclerosis). A fatty (cholesterol) material collects in an artery, narrowing it and eventually blocking the flow of blood.

All the following **adjective suffixes** mean "pertaining to" and *describe* a part of the body, process, or condition.

-al or -eal	pertaining to	peritone**al** _____
		inguin**al** _____
		ren**al** _____
		esophag**eal** _____
		myocardi**al** _____ A heart attack is also called a *myocardial infarction.* An infarction is an area of dead tissue caused by ischemia (when blood supply is held back from a part of the body).
-ar	pertaining to	vascul**ar** _____ A *cerebrovascular accident* is a stroke.
-ary	pertaining to	axill**ary** _____
		mamm**ary** _____
-ic	pertaining to	chron**ic** _____ Chronic conditions occur over a long period of time, as opposed to *acute* conditions, which are sharp, sudden, and brief.
		pelv**ic** _____

Procedural Suffixes

The following suffixes describe *procedures* used in patient care.

Suffix	*Meaning*	*Terminology*	*Meaning*
-centesis	surgical puncture to remove fluid	thoraco**centesis** _____ Also called *thoracentesis.* See Figure 3–5, next page.	
		amnio**centesis** _____ See Figure 3–6.	
		arthro**centesis** _____	

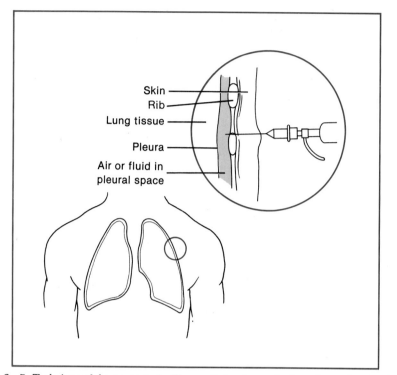

Figure 3–5. Technique of thoracocentesis. The needle is advanced only as far as the pleural space.

| -ectomy | removal, resection, excision | tonsillectomy _____
Tonsils and adenoids are *lymph tissue* in the throat. Lymph is composed of white blood cells that fight infection. See Figure 3–7.

hysterectomy _____
In a *total* hysterectomy, the whole uterus, including the cervix, is removed. If a portion of the uterus is not removed, the procedure is termed a *partial* or *subtotal* hysterectomy. See Figure 3–8.

oophorectomy _____

salpingectomy _____

cholecystectomy _____
See Figure 3–9.

mastectomy _____
Table 3–2 lists additional resection procedures. |

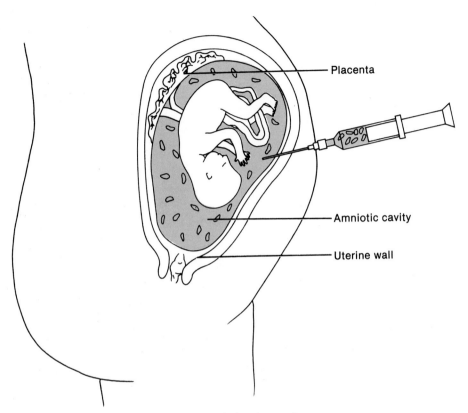

Placenta

Amniotic cavity

Uterine wall

Figure 3 – 6. Amniocentesis.

Figure 3 – 7. Tonsils and Adenoids.

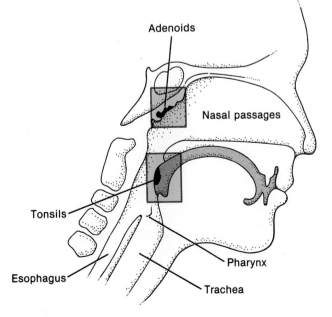

Adenoids

Nasal passages

Tonsils

Esophagus

Pharynx

Trachea

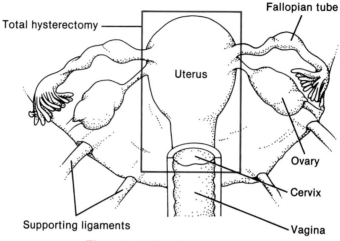

Figure 3–8. Total hysterectomy.

-gram	record

myelogram _____

MYEL/O means "spinal cord" in this term. A dye is injected into the membranes around the spinal cord (by *lumbar puncture*), and then x-ray pictures are taken of the spinal cord. Figure 3–10 shows a lumbar puncture.

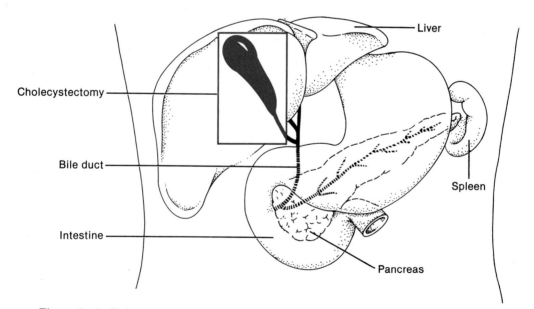

Figure 3–9. Cholecystectomy. The liver is lifted up to show the gallbladder underneath it. The pancreas is a long, thin gland located behind and to the left of the stomach, toward the spleen.

Table 3–2.   Resections

appendectomy	Excision of the appendix
adenectomy	Excision of a gland
adenoidectomy	Excision of the adenoids
colectomy	Excision of the colon
gastrectomy	Excision of the stomach
laminectomy	Excision of a piece of backbone (lamina) to relieve pressure on nerves from a (herniating) disk
lobectomy	Excision of a lobe of the lung
myomectomy	Excision of a muscle tumor
splenectomy	Excision of the spleen

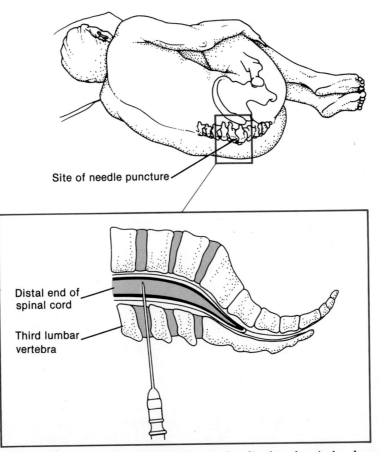

Site of needle puncture

Distal end of
spinal cord

Third lumbar
vertebra

Figure 3–10. Lumbar puncture. The distal end of the spinal cord is where the spinal cord nerves begin to fan out towards the legs. The lumbar puncture (spinal tap) is made below this area to avoid injuring the spinal cord. Fluid can be injected or withdrawn through the needle.

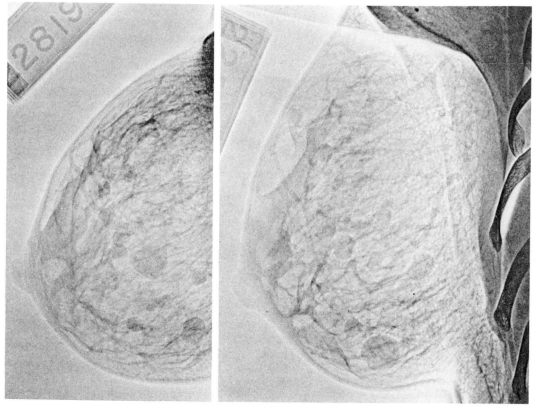

Figure 3–11. Mammograms. Fibrocystic (sacs of fluid and fibrous tissue) masses can be seen in both breasts.

		mammogram _____
		See Figure 3–11.
-graphy	process of recording	electroencephalography _____
		angiography _____
-lysis	separation, breakdown, destruction	dialysis _____

Hemodialysis is the removal of blood and its passage through a kidney machine to filter out waste materials, such as *urea*. Another form of dialysis is *peritoneal* dialysis. A special fluid is put into the peritoneum through a tube in the abdomen. The wastes seep into the fluid from the blood during a period of time. The fluid and wastes are then drained from the peritoneum. See Figure 3–12.

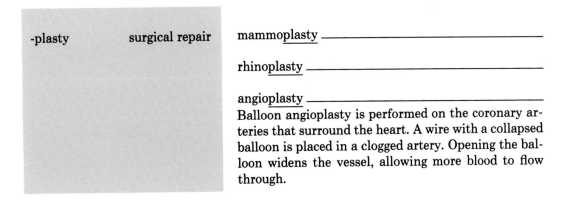

-plasty	surgical repair

mammoplasty _____

rhinoplasty _____

angioplasty _____
Balloon angioplasty is performed on the coronary arteries that surround the heart. A wire with a collapsed balloon is placed in a clogged artery. Opening the balloon widens the vessel, allowing more blood to flow through.

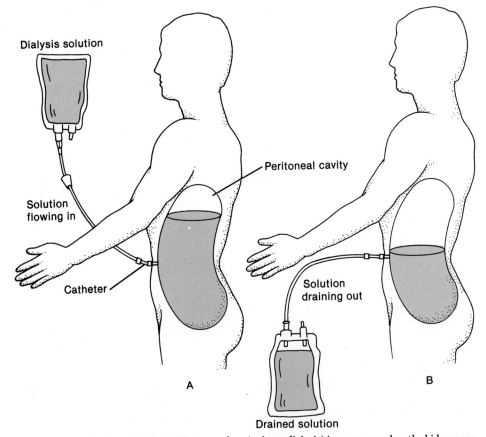

Dialysis solution

Solution flowing in

Catheter

Peritoneal cavity

Solution draining out

Drained solution

A   B

Figure 3–12. Peritoneal dialysis. This procedure (or hemodialysis) is necessary when the kidneys are not functioning to remove waste materials (such as urea) from the blood. Without dialysis or kidney transplantation, uremia can result.

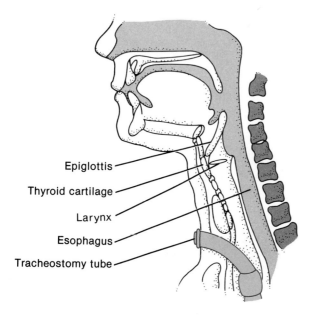

Figure 3–13. Tracheostomy, with tube in place.

Epiglottis

Thyroid cartilage

Larynx

Esophagus

Tracheostomy tube

-scopy	process of visual examination	arthroscopy _____
		laparoscopy _____
-stomy	opening	colostomy _____

A -STOMY procedure is the creation of a permanent or semipermanent opening from an organ to the outside of the body. STOMAT/O is a combining form for mouth.

tracheostomy _____
See Figure 3–13.

-therapy	treatment	radiotherapy _____
		chemotherapy _____
-tomy	incision, to cut into	craniotomy _____

-TOMY indicates a temporary incision, as opposed to -STOMY, which is a permanent or semipermanent opening.

laparotomy _____

IV. EXERCISES

A. *Match the following diagnostic suffixes in Column I with their meanings in Column II.*

Column I

1. -pathy   _____

2. -rrhea   _____

3. -algia   _____

4. -oma   _____

5. -itis   _____

6. -rrhagia   _____

7. -sclerosis _____

8. -osis   _____

9. -emia   _____

10. -megaly   _____

Column II

A. Hardening
B. Discharge, flow
C. Inflammation
D. Blood condition
E. Pain
F. Enlargement
G. Disease condition
H. Tumor, mass
I. Bursting forth of blood
J. Abnormal condition

Answer Key: 1. G   2. B   3. E   4. H   5. C   6. I   7. A   8. J
9. D   10. F

B. *Match the following procedural suffixes in Column I with their meanings in Column II.*

Column I

1. -tomy   _____

2. -scopy   _____

Column II

A. Removal, resection, excision
B. Visual examination
C. Process of recording
D. Opening

3. -therapy ——
E. Record
F. Separation, breakdown, destruction
4. -stomy ——
G. Treatment
H. Surgical repair
5. -lysis ——
I. Incision, to cut into
J. Surgical puncture to remove fluid
6. -centesis ——

7. -plasty ——

8. -graphy ——

9. -ectomy ——

10. -gram ——

Answer Key: 1. I   2. B   3. G   4. D   5. F   6. J   7. H   8. C
9. A   10. E

C. *Select from the following terms to complete the sentences below:*

myalgia	angioplasty	hematuria
septicemia	rhinorrhea	leukemia
thoracocentesis	menorrhagia	arteriosclerosis
laryngitis	esophagitis	ischemia

1. Surgical puncture to remove fluid from the chest is called _____

2. Surgical repair of a blood vessel is called _____

3. Muscle pain is called _____

4. Inflammation of the tube leading from the throat to the stomach is _____

5. Holding back blood from an organ or depriving it of blood supply is _____

6. Discharge of mucus from the nose is called _____

7. Blood in the urine is called _____

8. A malignant condition of increase in abnormal white blood cells is _____

9. Hardening of arteries is called _____

10. Excessive discharge of blood during menstruation is called _____

11. Inflammation of the voice box is known as _____

12. A blood infection is called _____

Answer Key: 1. thoracocentesis   2. angioplasty   3. myalgia   4. esophagitis   5. ischemia   6. rhinorrhea   7. hematuria   8. leukemia   9. arteriosclerosis   10. menorrhagia   11. laryngitis   12. septicemia

D. *Underline the suffix and give meanings for the following terms:*

1. bronchitis _____

2. encephalopathy _____

3. pelvic _____

4. carcinoma _____

5. chronic _____

6. otalgia _____

7. inguinal _____

8. mastectomy _____

9. colostomy _____

10. arthroscopy _____

11. cardiomegaly _____

12. hematuria _____

13. uremia _____

14. necrosis _____

Answer Key: 1. bronchitis—inflammation of bronchial tubes   2. encephalopathy —disease of the brain   3. pelvic—pertaining to the hip bone   4. carcinoma— cancerous tumor (of epithelial or skin tissue)   5. chronic—pertaining to occurring over a long period of time   6. otalgia—pain in the ear (earache)   7. inguinal— pertaining to the groin   8. mastectomy—removal of a breast   9. colostomy— opening of the colon to the outside of the body   10. arthroscopy—visual examination of a joint   11. cardiomegaly—enlargement of the heart 12. hematuria—blood in the urine   13. uremia—high levels of urea (waste material) in the blood   14. necrosis—abnormal condition of death of cells

E.   *Name the part of the body described in the following terms and give the meaning of each term:*

1.   cholecystectomy _____

2.   myalgia _____

3.   neuralgia _____

4.   nephrosis _____

5.   colitis _____

6.   myocardial ischemia _____

7.   renal _____

8.   hysterectomy _____

9.   laparoscopy _____

10.   mammoplasty _____

11.   axillary _____

12.   pneumonia _____

Answer Key: 1. gallbladder (removal of the gallbladder)   2. muscle (muscle pain)   3. nerve (nerve pain)   4. kidney (abnormal condition of a kidney)

5. colon (inflammation of the colon)   6. heart muscle (holding back blood to heart muscle)   7. kidney (pertaining to the kidney)   8. uterus (removal of the uterus)   9. abdomen (visual examination of the abdomen)   10. breast (surgical repair of the breast)   11. armpit (pertaining to the armpit)   12. lung (abnormal condition of the lung)

*F. **Match the following procedures with their meanings given below:***

radiotherapy	colostomy	craniotomy	rhinoplasty
amniocentesis	tracheostomy	electroencephalography	hemodialysis
laparoscopy	chemotherapy	myelogram	laparotomy

1. Treatment with drugs: _____

2. Surgical repair of the nose: _____

3. Separation of waste (urea) from the blood: _____

4. Opening of the windpipe to the outside of the body: _____

5. Surgical puncture to remove fluid from the sac around the fetus: _____

6. Incision of the skull: _____

7. Visual (endoscopic) examination of the abdomen: _____

8. Treatment with x-rays: _____

9. Record (x-ray) of the spinal cord: _____

10. Opening of the colon to the outside of the body: _____

11. Process of recording the electricity in the brain: _____

12. Incision of the abdomen (abdominal wall): _____

Answer Key: 1. chemotherapy   2. rhinoplasty   3. hemodialysis
4. tracheostomy   5. amniocentesis   6. craniotomy   7. laparoscopy
8. radiotherapy   9. myelogram   10. colostomy   11. electroencephalography
12. laparotomy

G. *Underline the correctly spelled terms and give their meanings.*

1.   myleogram   myelogram   _____

2.   peritoneal   peritonal   _____

3.   colocystitis   cholecystitis   _____

4.   chemotheraphy   chemotherapy   _____

5.   hemmorrage   hemorrhage   _____

6.   myalgia   myoalgia   _____

7.   tonsilectomy   tonsillectomy   _____

8.   -sclerosis   -sklerosis   _____

9.   arthraljia   arthralgia   _____

10.   larnyx   larynx   _____

11.   cardiomegaly   cardiomeagaly   _____

12.   oophorectomy   oopherectomy   _____

13.   meninjitis   meningitis   _____

14.   axillary   axillery   _____

15.   erythrocytosis   erithrocytosis   _____

Answer Key: 1. myelogram — x-ray record of the spinal cord   2. peritoneal — pertaining to the peritoneum (membrane around the abdominal organs)
3. cholecystitis — inflammation of the gallbladder   4. chemotherapy — treatment of disease with drugs   5. hemorrhage — bursting forth of blood   6. myalgia — muscle pain   7. tonsillectomy — removal of tonsils   8. -sclerosis — hardening   9. arthralgia — pain of joints   10. larynx — voice box
11. cardiomegaly — enlargement of the heart   12. oophorectomy — removal of an ovary   13. meningitis — inflammation of the meninges   14. axillary — pertaining to the armpit   15. erythrocytosis — abnormal condition (slight increase in numbers) of red blood cells

H. *Match the following abnormal conditions with their descriptions below:*

atherosclerosis   hematuria   septicemia   nephrosis
carcinoma   cardiomyopathy   sarcoma   adenoma
myocardial infarction   uremia   hepatomegaly   cerebrovascular accident

1. Malignant tumor of connective tissue: _____

2. Benign tumor of a gland: _____

3. Heart attack (area of dead tissue in heart muscle): _____

4. Hardening of arteries by collection of plaque: _____

5. Stroke (blood vessels in the brain are damaged): _____

6. Disease condition of heart muscle (not a heart attack): _____

7. Abnormal condition of the kidney: _____

8. Blood infection: _____

9. Blood in the urine: _____

10. Excessive urea in the blood: _____

11. Cancerous tumor (of epithelial or surface tissues): _____

12. Enlargement of the liver: _____

Answer Key: 1. sarcoma   2. adenoma   3. myocardial infarction
4. atherosclerosis   5. cerebrovascular accident   6. cardiomyopathy
7. nephrosis   8. septicemia   9. hematuria   10. uremia   11. carcinoma
12. hepatomegaly

I. *What part of the body is inflamed?*

1. neuritis _____

2. arthritis _____

3. salpingitis _____

4. otitis _____

5. hepatitis _____

6. nephritis _____

7. esophagitis _____

8. laryngitis _____

9. encephalitis _____

10. osteitis _____

11. meningitis _____

12. bronchitis _____

13. rhinitis _____

14. peritonitis _____

15. vasculitis _____

16. mastitis _____

17. tonsillitis _____

18. colitis _____

19. pharyngitis _____

20. tracheitis _____

J. *Provide the terms for the following procedures:*

1. Excision of the gallbladder _____

2. Excision of the appendix _____

3. Excision of a breast _____

4. Excision of the uterus _____

5. Excision of an ovary _____

6. Excision of the voice box _____

7. Excision of the kidney _____

8. Excision of a gland _____

9. Excision of the large intestine _____

10. Excision of a fallopian tube _____

11. Excision of tonsils _____

12. Incision of the skull _____

13. Incision of the abdomen _____

14. Incision of the chest _____

15. Opening of the windpipe to the outside of the body _____

16. Opening of the colon to the outside of the body _____

17. Surgical puncture of the chest _____

18. Surgical puncture of the sac around the fetus _____

Answer Key: 1. cholecystectomy   2. appendectomy   3. mastectomy
4. hysterectomy   5. oophorectomy   6. laryngectomy   7. nephrectomy
8. adenectomy   9. colectomy   10. salpingectomy   11. tonsillectomy
12. craniotomy   13. laparotomy   14. thoracotomy   15. tracheostomy
16. colostomy   17. thoracentesis or thoracocentesis   18. amniocentesis

K. **Select from the following to complete the following definitions:**

adenoma	adenocarcinoma	osteoma	arthropathy
hepatoma	myoma	hematoma	cardiomyopathy
radiotherapy	myosarcoma	encephalopathy	neuropathy

1.   Collection (mass) of blood _____

2.   Tumor of muscle (benign) _____

3.   Treatment using x-rays _____

4.   Tumor of a gland (benign) _____

5.   Tumor of bone (benign) _____

6.   Cancerous tumor of glandular tissue _____

7.   Malignant tumor (flesh tissue) of muscle _____

8.   Tumor of the liver _____

9.   Disease of joints _____

10.   Disease of heart muscle _____

11.   Disease of nerves _____

12.   Disease of the brain _____

Answer Key: 1. hematoma   2. myoma   3. radiotherapy   4. adenoma
5. osteoma   6. adenocarcinoma   7. myosarcoma   8. hepatoma
9. arthropathy   10. cardiomyopathy   11. neuropathy   12. encephalopathy

V.   REVIEW

Write the meanings for the following word parts, and don't forget to check your answers.

SUFFIXES

Suffixes	Meanings		Suffixes	Meanings
1. -al	_____		3. -ar	_____
2. -algia	_____		4. -ary	_____

Suffixes	Meanings		Suffixes	Meanings
5. -centesis	_____		17. -osis	_____
6. -eal	_____		18. -pathy	_____
7. -ectomy	_____		19. -plasty	_____
8. -emia	_____		20. -rrhage	_____
9. -gram	_____		21. -rrhagia	_____
10. -graphy	_____		22. -rrhea	_____
11. -ia	_____		23. -sclerosis	_____
12. -ic	_____		24. -scopy	_____
13. -itis	_____		25. -stomy	_____
14. -lysis	_____		26. -therapy	_____
15. -megaly	_____		27. -tomy	_____
16. -oma	_____		28. -uria	_____

COMBINING FORMS

Combining Forms	Meanings		Combining Forms	Meanings
1. aden/o	_____		9. carcin/o	_____
2. amni/o	_____		10. cardi/o	_____
3. angi/o	_____		11. chem/o	_____
4. arteri/o	_____		12. cholecyst/o	_____
5. arthr/o	_____		13. chron/o	_____
6. ather/o	_____		14. col/o	_____
7. axill/o	_____		15. crani/o	_____
8. bronch/o	_____		16. cyst/o	_____

Combining Forms	Meanings		Combining Forms	Meanings
17. encephal/o	_____		36. neur/o	_____
18. erythr/o	_____		37. oophor/o	_____
19. esophag/o	_____		38. oste/o	_____
20. hemat/o	_____		39. ot/o	_____
21. hepat/o	_____		40. pelv/o	_____
22. hyster/o	_____		41. peritone/o	_____
23. inguin/o	_____		42. pneumon/o	_____
24. isch/o	_____		43. radi/o	_____
25. lapar/o	_____		44. ren/o	_____
26. laryng/o	_____		45. rhin/o	_____
27. leuk/o	_____		46. salping/o	_____
28. mamm/o	_____		47. sarc/o	_____
29. mast/o	_____		48. septic/o	_____
30. men/o	_____		49. thorac/o	_____
31. mening/o	_____		50. tonsill/o	_____
32. my/o	_____		51. trache/o	_____
33. myel/o	_____		52. ur/o	_____
34. necr/o	_____		53. vascul/o	_____
35. nephr/o	_____			

SUFFIXES

Answer Key: 1. pertaining to   2. pain   3. pertaining to   4. pertaining to   5. surgical puncture to remove fluid   6. pertaining to   7. removal, resection, excision   8. blood condition   9. record   10. process of recording   11. condition   12. pertaining to   13. inflammation   14. separation, breakdown, destruction   15. enlargement   16. tumor, mass   17. abnormal condition   18. disease condition   19. surgical repair   20. bursting forth of blood   21. bursting forth of blood   22. flow, discharge   23. hardening   24. visual examination   25. opening   26. treatment   27. incision   28. urine condition

COMBINING FORMS

Answer Key: 1. gland   2. amnion   3. blood vessel   4. artery   5. joint   6. plaque, collection of fatty material   7. armpit   8. bronchial tubes   9. cancerous   10. heart   11. drug, chemical   12. gallbladder   13. time   14. colon (large intestine)   15. skull   16. urinary bladder   17. brain   18. red   19. esophagus   20. blood   21. liver   22. uterus   23. groin   24. to hold back   25. abdomen   26. larynx (voice box)   27. white   28. breast   29. breast   30. menstruation   31. meninges   32. muscle   33. spinal cord or bone marrow   34. death   35. kidney   36. nerve   37. ovary   38. bone   39. ear   40. hip bone   41. peritoneum   42. lungs   43. x-rays   44. kidney   45. nose   46. fallopian tube   47. flesh   48. pertaining to infection   49. chest   50. tonsils   51. trachea (windpipe)   52. urine, urinary tract   53. blood vessel

---

VI.   PRONUNCIATION OF TERMS

Write the meaning of each term next to its pronunciation.

Term	Pronunciation	Meaning
adenocarcinoma	ah-deh-no-kar-sih-**NO**-mah	_____
adenoma	ah-deh-**NO**-mah	_____
amniocentesis	am-ne-o-sen-**TE**-sis	_____

angioplasty	**AN**-je-o-plas-te ———————————————
arteriosclerosis	ar-ter-i-o-skle-**RO**-sis ———————————
arthralgia	ar-**THRAL**-je-ah ———————————————
arthropathy	ar-**THROP**-ah-the ———————————————
arthroscopy	ar-**THROS**-ko-pe ———————————————
atherosclerosis	ah-theh-ro-skle-**RO**-sis ————————————
axillary	**AKS**-ih-lar-e ———————————————————
bronchitis	brong-**KI**-tis ————————————————————
carcinoma	kar-sih-**NO**-mah ———————————————
cardiomegaly	kar-de-o-**MEG**-ah-le ———————————
cardiomyopathy	kar-de-o-mi-**OP**-ah-the ————————
chemotherapy	ke-mo-**THER**-ah-pe ———————————
cholecystectomy	ko-le-sis-**TEK**-to-me ———————————
chronic	**KRON**-ik ———————————————————
colitis	ko-**LI**-tis —————————————————————
colostomy	ko-**LOS**-to-me ———————————————
craniotomy	kra-ne-**OT**-o-me ———————————————
cystitis	sis-**TI**-tis ———————————————————
dialysis	di-**AL**-ih-sis ———————————————————
electroencephalography	e-lek-tro-en-sef-ah-**LOG**-rah-fe ———————
encephalopathy	en-sef-ah-**LOP**-ah-the —————————
erythrocytosis	eh-rith-ro-si-**TO**-sis ———————————
esophageal	e-sof-ah-**JE**-al ———————————————

esophagitis	e-sof-ah-**JI**-tis _____
hematoma	he-mah-**TO**-mah _____
hematuria	he-mah-**TUR**-e-ah _____
hemorrhage	**HEM**-or-ij _____
hysterectomy	his-teh-**REK**-to-me _____
infarction	in-**FARK**-shun _____
inguinal	**ING**-gwi-nal _____
ischemia	is-**KE**-me-ah _____
laparoscopy	lap-ah-**ROS**-ko-pe _____
laparotomy	lap-ah-**ROT**-o-me _____
laryngitis	lah-rin-**JI**-tis _____
leukemia	lu-**KE**-me-ah _____
mammogram	**MAM**-o-gram _____
mammography	ma-**MOG**-rah-fe _____
mammoplasty	**MAM**-o-plas-te _____
mastectomy	mas-**TEK**-to-me _____
meningitis	men-in-**JI**-tis _____
menorrhagia	men-or-**RA**-jah/men-or-**RA**-je-ah _____
menorrhea	men-o-**RE**-ah _____
myalgia	mi-**AL**-je-ah _____
myelogram	**MI**-eh-lo-gram _____
myocardial	mi-o-**KAR**-de-al _____
myoma	mi-**O**-mah _____

myosarcoma	mi-o-sar-**KO**-mah _____
necrosis	neh-**KRO**-sis _____
nephrosis	neh-**FRO**-sis _____
neuralgia	nu-**RAL**-je-ah _____
oophorectomy	o-of-o-**REK**-to-me/oo-for-**REK**-to-me _____
otalgia	o-**TAL**-je-ah _____
pelvic	**PEL**-vik _____
peritoneal	per-ih-to-**NE**-al _____
radiotherapy	ra-de-o-**THER**-ah-pe _____
renal	**RE**-nal _____
rhinoplasty	**RI**-no-plas-te _____
rhinorrhea	ri-no-**RE**-ah _____
salpingectomy	sal-ping-**JEK**-to-me _____
sarcoma	sar-**KO**-mah _____
septic	**SEP**-tik _____
septicemia	sep-ti-**SE**-me-ah _____
thoracentesis	tho-rah-sen-**TE**-sis _____
thoracocentesis	tho-rah-ko-sen-**TE**-sis _____
tonsillectomy	ton-si-**LEK**-to-me _____
tracheostomy	tra-ke-**OS**-to-me _____
uremia	u-**RE**-me-ah _____
vascular	**VAS**-ku-lar _____

CHAPTER 4

PREFIXES

CHAPTER SECTIONS

CHAPTER OBJECTIVES

- To identify and define commom prefixes used in medical terms
- To analyze, spell, and pronounce medical terms that contain prefixes

I. INTRODUCTION

This chapter includes prefixes that were introduced in Chapter 1 and adds new prefixes as well. The list of combining forms and suffixes in Section II helps you understand the terminology in Section III. Complete the exercises in Section IV and the review in Section V. Don't forget to check your answers! The answers to exercises are placed directly after the questions so that you can use them easily. The pronunciation list in Section VI is your final review of the terminology in this chapter.

II. COMBINING FORMS AND SUFFIXES

Combining Form	Meaning
abdomin/o	abdomen
an/o	anus (opening of the digestive tract to the outside of the body)
bi/o	life
cardi/o	heart
carp/o	carpals (wrist bones)
cis/o	to cut
cost/o	ribs
crani/o	skull
cutane/o	skin
dur/o	dura mater (outermost meningeal membrane surrounding the brain and spinal cord)
gen/o	to produce, to begin
glyc/o	sugar
hemat/o	blood
later/o	side
men/o	menses (monthly discharge of blood from the lining of the uterus)
nat/i	birth
norm/o	rule, order
oste/o	bone
peritone/o	peritoneum (membrane surrounding the organs in the abdomen)
plas/o	formation, growth, development
ren/o	kidney
scapul/o	scapula (shoulder blade)
son/o	sound
thyroid/o	thyroid gland
top/o	to put, place, position
troph/o	development, nourishment
urethr/o	urethra (tube leading from the bladder to the outside of the body)

uter/o	uterus
ven/o	vein
vertebr/o	vertebra (backbone)

Suffix	*Meaning*
-al	pertaining to
-ation	process, condition
-cision	process of cutting
-crine	secretion
-emia	blood condition
-gen	to produce
-graphy	process of recording
-ia	condition, process
-ic	pertaining to
-ine	pertaining to
-ism	condition, process
-lapse	to fall, slide
-lysis	loosening, breakdown, separation, destruction
-mission	to send
-mortem	death
-oma	tumor, mass
-ous	pertaining to
-partum	birth
-plasm	formation
-pnea	breathing
-rrhea	flow, discharge
-scopy	process of visual examination
-section	to cut
-stasis	stop, control
-tension	pressure
-thesis	to put, place
-tic	pertaining to
-um	structure
-uria	urine condition
-y	process, condition

III. PREFIXES AND TERMINOLOGY

Prefix	*Meaning*	*Terminology*	*Meaning*
a-, an-	no, not, without	apnea _____	

Table 4–1. Anemias

aplastic anemia	Bone marrow fails to produce red blood cells (erythrocytes), white blood cells (leukocytes), and clotting cells (platelets).
hemolytic anemia	Red blood cells are destroyed (-lytic), and bone marrow cannot compensate for their loss. This condition can be hereditary or acquired (after infection or chemotherapy) or can occur when the immune system acts against normal red blood cells (autoimmune condition).
iron deficiency anemia	Low or absent iron levels lead to low hemoglobin concentration or deficiency of red blood cells.
pernicious anemia	The mucous membrane of the stomach fails to produce a factor (intrinsic factor) that is necessary for the absorption of vitamin B_{12} and the proper formation of red blood cells.
sickle cell anemia	Erythrocytes assume an abnormal crescent or sickle shape; it is caused by the inheritance of an abnormal type of hemoglobin. The sickle-shaped cells clump together, causing clots that block blood vessels.

<u>a</u>trophy _____
Muscular atrophy can occur because of disuse of the muscle.

<u>a</u>nemia _____
Anemia is a lower number of red blood cells or a decrease in hemoglobin in the cells. Table 4–1 lists some of the different forms of anemia.

<u>a</u>menorrhea _____

ab-	away from	<u>ab</u>normal _____
ad-	toward, near	<u>ad</u>renal glands _____ See Figure 4–1.
ana-	up, apart	<u>ana</u>lysis _____ A *urinalysis* (urine + analysis) is a separation of urine to determine its parts.
ante-	before, forward	<u>ante</u> partum _____ <u>ante</u> mortem _____
anti-	against	<u>anti</u>bodies _____ Antibodies are proteins that are made by white blood cells; literally, they are "bodies" that are "against" foreign substances.

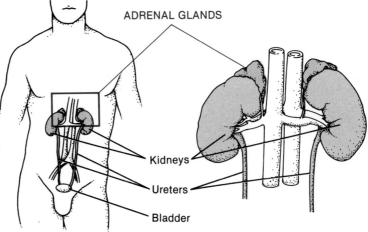

ADRENAL GLANDS

Kidneys

Ureters

Bladder

FIGURE 4–1. Adrenal glands. These two endocrine glands are above each kidney.

antigen _____
Antigens are foreign substances, such as bacteria and viruses. When antigens enter the body, they stimulate white blood cells to produce antibodies that act against the antigens. Think of the ANTI in *antigen* as standing for antibody, so that *antigen* means "to produce (-gen) antibodies."

antibiotic _____
Antibiotics differ from antibodies in that they are produced *outside* the body by primitive plants called molds. Examples of antibiotics are penicillin and erythromycin.

bi-	two, both	bilateral _____
brady-	slow	bradycardia _____
con-	with, together	congenital _____

congenital _____
A congenital anomaly is an irregularity (anomaly) that a person is born with. Examples are webbed fingers and toes and heart defects.

dia- | through, complete

diarrhea _____

dialysis _____

-LYSIS means "separation" here.

dys-	bad, painful	dyspnea _____
		dysplasia _____
	difficult	dysmenorrhea _____
		dysuria _____
ec-	out, outside	ectopic pregnancy _____

Figure 4–2 shows possible sites of ectopic pregnancies.

| endo- | within, in, inner | endoscopy _____ |

Table 4–2 lists examples of endoscopies.

endocrine glands _____

The adrenal glands are endocrine glands.

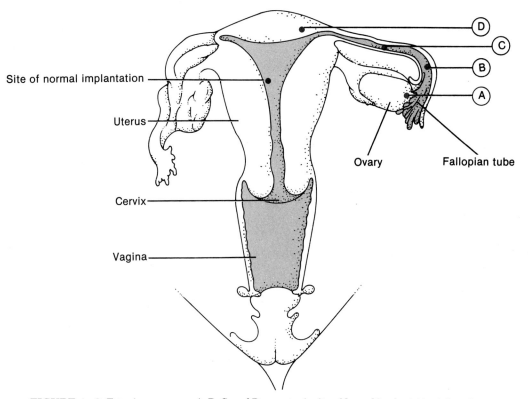

FIGURE 4–2. Ectopic pregnancy. A, B, C, and D are ectopic sites. Normal implantation takes place on the inner lining (endometrium) of the uterus.

Table 4–2.   Endoscopies

arthroscopy	Visual examination of a joint
bronchoscopy	Visual examination of the bronchial tubes
colonoscopy	Visual examination of the colon (large intestine)
cystoscopy	Visual examination of the urinary bladder
esophagoscopy	Visual examination of the esophagus
gastroscopy	Visual examination of the stomach
hysteroscopy	Visual examination of the uterus
laparoscopy	Visual examination of the abdomen
laryngoscopy	Visual examination of the larynx (voice box)
mediastinoscopy	Visual examination of the mediastinum
proctosigmoidoscopy	Visual examination of the rectum and sigmoid colon
sigmoidoscopy	Visual examination of the sigmoid colon (lower, S-shaped part of the large intestine)

epi-	above, upon	epidural hematoma _____ Figure 4–3 illustrates epidural and subdural hematomas.
		epidermis _____ The three layers of the skin, from outermost to innermost, are the epidermis, dermis, and subcutaneous layer. Check *Appendix I* (Skin and Sense Organs) for a diagram of the skin.
ex-	out	excision _____
extra-	outside of	extrahepatic _____
hyper-	excessive, above	hyperthyroidism _____ Figure 4–4 shows the position of the thyroid gland in the neck.
		hypertrophy _____ Cells increase in size, not in number. The opposite of hypertrophy is *atrophy* (cells shrink in size).
		hypertension _____ Risk factors that contribute to high blood pressure are increasing age, smoking, obesity, heredity, and a stressful life style.
		hyperglycemia _____ Also known as diabetes mellitus. *Mellitus* means "sweet."

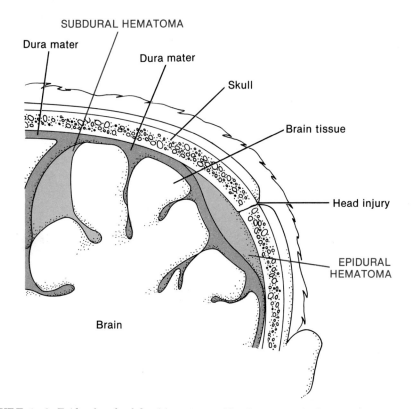

FIGURE 4-3. Epidural and subdural hematomas. The dura mater is the outermost of the three meninges (membranes) around the brain and spinal cord.

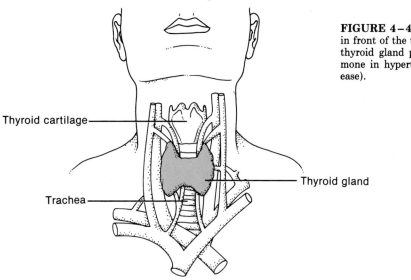

FIGURE 4-4. Thyroid gland, located in front of the trachea in the neck. The thyroid gland produces too much hormone in hyperthyroidism (Graves' disease).

hypo-	below, deficient	hypoglycemia _____
in-	in, into	incision _____
inter-	between	intervertebral _____
intra-	within	intrauterine _____
		intravenous _____
mal-	bad	malignant _____

mal- | bad

malignant _____

-IGNANT comes from the Latin *ignis* meaning a "fire." A malignant tumor is a cancerous tumor. A *benign* tumor (*ben* means "good") is a non-cancerous growth.

meta- | beyond

metastasis _____

This term literally means "beyond control." It is the spread of a cancerous tumor from its original location to a secondary place in the body.

metacarpals _____

The carpal bones are the wrist bones, and the metacarpals are the hand bones, which are "beyond the wrist." See the x-ray picture of the hand in Figure 4–5.

neo- | new

neoplasm _____

neoplastic _____

neonatal _____

para- | near, along the side of

parathyroid glands _____

Figure 4–6 shows the position of the parathyroid glands on the back side of the thyroid gland. The parathyroid glands are endocrine glands that regulate the amount of calcium in bones and in the blood.

paralysis _____

This term came from the Greek *paralyikos*, meaning "one whose side was loose or weak," as after a stroke. Now it means a loss of movement in any part of the body caused by a break in the connection between nerve and muscle.

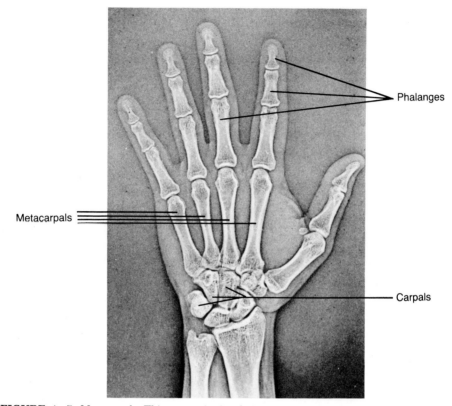

FIGURE 4–5. Metacarpals. This x-ray of a hand shows metacarpals, carpals (wrist bones) and phalanges (finger bones).

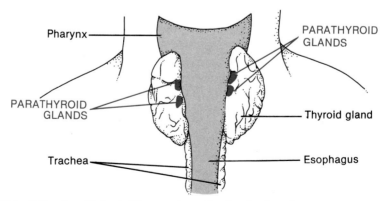

FIGURE 4–6. Parathyroid glands. These are four endocrine glands on the posterior (back side) of the thyroid gland.

peri-	surrounding	periosteum _____
		perianal _____
poly-	many, much	polyuria _____
post-	after, behind	post partum _____
		post mortem _____
pre-	before	precancerous _____
		prenatal _____
pro-	before, forward	prolapse _____
		-LAPSE means "to slide." Figure 4–7 shows a prolapsed uterus.
pros-	before, forward	prosthesis _____
		An artificial limb is a prosthesis. Figure 4–8 illustrates several types of prostheses.
re-	back, behind	relapse _____
		Symptoms of disease return.
		remission _____
		Symptoms of disease lessen.
		resection _____

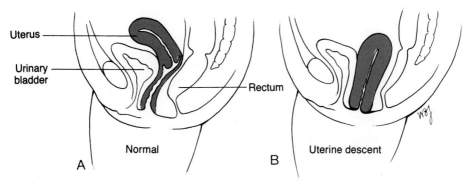

FIGURE 4–7. Prolapsed uterus is shown in (B). Normally the uterus is tilted forward above the bladder (A).

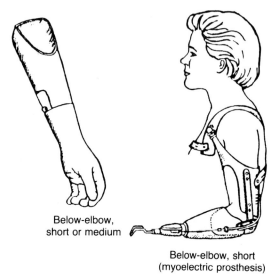

Below-elbow,
short or medium

Below-elbow, short
(myoelectric prosthesis)

FIGURE 4–8. Upper limb prostheses.

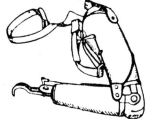

Above-elbow,
medium or long

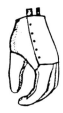

Artificial hand

retro-	back, behind	retroperitoneal _____ The kidneys and adrenal glands are retroperitoneal organs.
sub-	beneath, less than	subcostal _____
		subcutaneous _____
		subtotal _____ A subtotal gastrectomy is a partial resection of the stomach.
		subscapular _____ The scapula is the shoulder bone. Figure 4–9 shows its location.

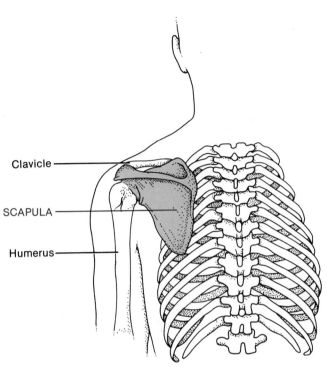

FIGURE 4–9. Scapula (shoulder bone), posterior view. The clavicle is the collar bone and the humerus is the upper arm bone.

Clavicle

SCAPULA

Humerus

syn-	with, together

syndrome _____
-DROME means "to run" or "occur." Syndromes are groups of symptoms or signs of illness that occur together. Table 4–3 gives examples of syndromes.

Table 4–3.   Syndromes

Acquired immune deficiency syndrome (AIDS)
Symptoms are severe infections, malignancy (Kaposi's sarcoma and lymphoma), fever, malaise (discomfort), and gastrointestinal disturbances. It is caused by a virus that damages lymphocytes (white blood cells).

Barlow's syndrome (mitral valve prolapse)
Symptoms are abnormal sounds (murmurs) heard from the chest when listening with a stethoscope. These murmurs indicate that the mitral valve is not closing properly. Chest pain, dyspnea (difficult breathing), and fatigue are other symptoms.

Carpal tunnel syndrome
Symptoms are pain, tingling, burning, and numbness of the hand. A nerve leading to the hand is compressed by connective tissue fibers in the wrist.

Down syndrome
Symptoms include mental retardation, flat face with a short nose, slanted eyes, broad hands and feet, stubby fingers, and protruding lower lip. The syndrome occurs when an extra chromosome is present in each cell of the body.

Toxic shock syndrome
Symptoms are high fever, vomiting, diarrhea, rash, hypotension (low blood pressure), and shock. It is caused by a bacterial infection in the vagina of menstruating women using superabsorbent tampons.

tachy-	fast	tachycardia _____
		tachypnea _____
trans-	across, through	transabdominal _____
		transurethral _____
tri-	three	tricuspid valve_____

CUSPID means "pointed end," as of a spear. The tricuspid valve is on the right side of the heart. The mitral or bicuspid valve is on the left side of the heart. Figure 4–10 shows the location of both valves and indicates the pathway of blood through the heart.

ultra-   beyond   ultrasonography _____

Figure 4–11 shows an ultrasonogram (sonogram) of a 30-week fetus.

uni-   one   unilateral _____

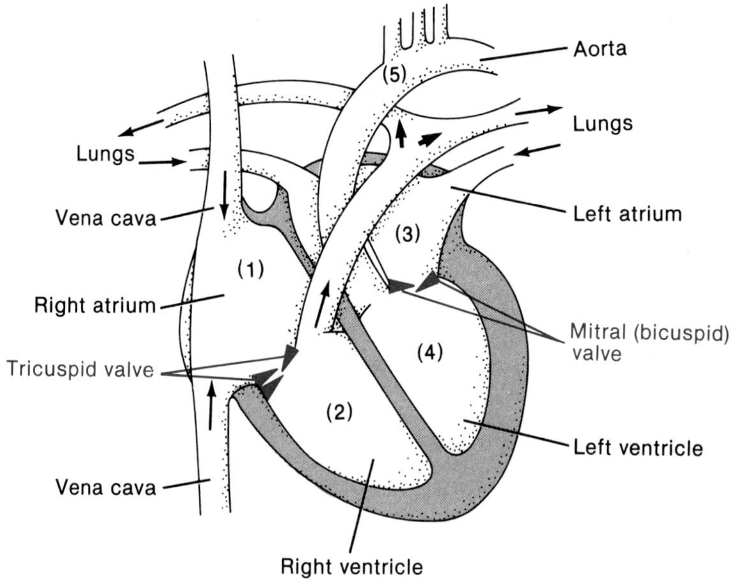

FIGURE 4–10. Tricuspid and mitral valves of the heart. Blood enters the *right atrium* of the heart (1) from the big veins (venae cavae) and passes through the *tricuspid valve* to the right ventricle (2). Blood then travels to the *lungs* where it loses carbon dioxide (a gaseous waste) and picks up oxygen. Blood returns to the heart into the *left atrium* (3) and passes through the mitral (bicuspid) valve to the *left ventricle* (4). It is then pumped from the left ventricle out the heart into the largest artery, the *aorta* (5), which carries the blood to all parts of the body.

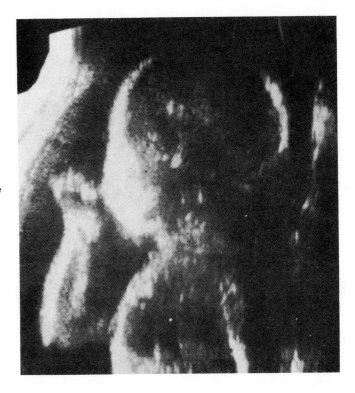

FIGURE 4–11. Ultrasonography. The 30-week fetus is sucking its thumb.

IV. EXERCISES

A. *Match the prefix in Column I with its meaning in Column II:*

Column I

1. dia- _____
2. neo- _____
3. peri- _____
4. an- _____
5. brady- _____
6. uni- _____
7. trans- _____

Column II

a. across, through
b. no, not, without
c. bad, painful, difficult
d. new
e. near, along the side of
f. surrounding
g. through, complete
h. one
i. slow
j. beyond

8. ultra- _____

9. para- _____

10. dys- _____

B. *Give meanings for the following prefixes:*

1. meta- _____

2. ana- _____

3. a-, an- _____

4. bi- _____

5. inter- _____

6. para- _____

7. in- _____

8. mal- _____

9. anti- _____

10. con- _____

C. **Select from the prefixes given in Column II to match meanings in Column I. Write the prefix in the space provided next to its meaning.**

Column I		Column II
1. bad, painful, difficult	_____	hyper-
		meta-
2. out, outside	_____	pro-, pros-
		intra-
3. away from	_____	syn-
		ab-
4. fast	_____	re-, retro-
		hypo-
5. before, forward	_____	uni-
		dia-
6. back, behind	_____	tachy-
		ec-
7. less than, below	_____	dys-
		ad-
8. three	_____	inter-
		tri-
9. together, with	_____	
10. within	_____	

Answer Key: 1. dys-   2. ec-   3. ab-   4. tachy-   5. pro-, pros-
6. re-, retro-   7. hypo-   8. tri-   9. syn-   10. intra-

D. **Give meanings for the following prefixes:**

1. ante- _____

2. ad- _____

3. brady- _____

4. endo- _____

5. epi- _____

6. post- _____

7. pre- _____

8. sub- _____

9. extra- _____

10. dia- _____

> **Answer Key:** 1. before, forward   2. toward   3. slow   4. within, in, inner   5. above, upon   6. after, behind   7. before   8. beneath, less than   9. out, outside of   10. through, complete

E. *Circle the meaning that is correct in each of the following:*

1. Dys- and mal- both mean (outside, good, bad).
2. Hypo- and sub- both mean (below, above, outside).
3. Epi- and hyper- both mean (inside, beneath, above).
4. Con- and syn- both mean (apart, near, with).
5. Ultra- and meta- both mean (new, beyond, without).
6. Ante-, pre-, and pro- all mean (before, surrounding, between).
7. Ec- and extra- both mean (within, many, outside).
8. Endo-, intra-, and in- all mean (painful, within, through).
9. Post-, re-, and retro- all mean (behind, slow, together).
10. Uni- means (one, two, three).
11. Tri- means (one, two, three).
12. Bi-means (three, one, two).

> **Answer Key:** 1. bad   2. below   3. above   4. with   5. beyond   6. before   7. outside   8. within   9. behind   10. one   11. three   12. two

F. *Select from the following terms to complete the sentences below. The words in italics should be clues in your choice of the correct terms.*

analysis	prenatal	atrophy	unilateral
dysmenorrhea	bradycardia	adrenal glands	extracranial
antibody	dyspnea	parathyroid glands	epidural hematoma
bilateral	metacarpal	hypertrophy	

1. Two glands located *near* (toward) the kidneys are the _____.

2. People suffering from asthma often have *difficult* breathing, known as _____.

3. A problem that only affects *one* side of the body is a(an) _____ defect.

4. Some people have a *slow* heart rhythm called _____.

5. A condition of *painful* menstrual discharge is called _____.

6. The bones that are *beyond* the wrist are the hand bones, or _____ bones.

7. A protein substance that is made by white blood cells *against* foreign microorganisms is

    called a(an) _____ .

8. An injury to the *outside* of the skull would be known as a(an) _____ lesion.

9. Four glands located in the neck region *near* another gland are _____.

10. Taking a substance *apart* to understand what it contains is called a(an) _____.

11. A collection of blood located *above* the outermost layer of membranes surrounding the

    brain is called a(an) _____.

12. A problem that occurs *before* the birth of an infant is called _____.

13. *Excessive* development (individual cells increase in size) of an organ is known as

    _____.

14. When a part of the body is not used, *no* development occurs, and it shrinks in size, known

    as _____.

15. A problem affecting *both* sides of the body is called a (an) _____ defect.

G. *Underline the prefix in each term, and give the meaning of the entire term:*

1. dysuria _____

2. hypoglycemia _____

3. intravenous _____

4. syndrome _____

5. precancerous _____

6. apnea _____

7. anemia _____

8. endoscopy _____

9. prosthesis _____

10. antibiotic _____

Answer Key: 1. <u>dys</u>uria — painful urination   2. <u>hypo</u>glycemia — low levels of sugar in the blood   3. <u>intra</u>venous — pertaining to within a vein   4. <u>syn</u>drome — group of symptoms that occur together, characterizing an abnormal condition   5. <u>pre</u>cancerous — before cancer   6. <u>a</u>pnea — not breathing   7. <u>an</u>emia — literally, no blood; actually a decrease in red blood cells or in the hemoglobin within the cells   8. <u>endo</u>scopy — process of viewing within the body (an endoscope is used)   9. <u>pros</u>thesis — to put or place before (an artificial body part)   10. <u>anti</u>biotic — pertaining to a substance that is against bacterial or germ life

H. *Define the following terms that describe an organ, tissue, or space in the body:*

1. subscapular _____

2. intrauterine _____

3. periosteum _____

4. intervertebral _____

5. subcostal _____

6. transabdominal _____

7. perianal _____

8. extracranial _____

9. subcutaneous _____

10. retroperitoneal _____

Answer Key: 1. under the shoulder   2. within the uterus   3. surrounding the bone (this is a membrane surrounding the bone)   4. between a vertebra (a disk is an intervertebral structure)   5. under a rib   6. across the abdomen   7. surrounding the anus   8. outside the skull   9. under the skin   10. behind the peritoneum

I.   Use the following terms to fill in the blanks in the sentences below:

congenital	ectopic	subtotal	metastasis
transurethral	prosthesis	malignant	hyperthyroidism
tachycardia	ultrasonography	tricuspid	endocrine
dialysis	diarrhea	dysplasia	antigen

1. Enlargement of an endocrine gland in the neck can lead to _____.

2. An artificial limb is a(an) _____.

3. If the colon does not reabsorb the proper amount of water back into the bloodstream,

    _____ occurs.

4. An abnormally rapid heart beat is a _____.

5. Infection or abnormal ("bad") growth of cells on the uterine cervix can cause a condition known as cervical _____.

6. A test that shows the structure of organs in the abdomen by using sound waves is _____.

7. The spread of a cancerous tumor to a secondary place in the body is a(an) _____.

8. The process of filtering the waste materials from the blood using a machine that does the work of the kidneys is called _____.

9. The _____ valve is composed of three points and is located on the right side of the heart between the upper and lower chambers.

10. A procedure to remove the prostate gland by cutting across (through) the urethra is a _____ resection of the prostate.

11. Cancerous growths are _____ neoplasms.

12. An abnormal condition that occurs at birth is a(an) _____ anomaly.

13. A gland that secretes hormones into the bloodstream is a(an) _____ gland.

14. A foreign organism, such as a virus or bacterium, that enters the body and stimulates white blood cells to make antibodies, is a(an) _____.

15. An embryo that grows outside the uterus (extrauterine) is a(an) _____ pregnancy.

16. The doctors did not remove the whole organ; they did a(an) _____ resection.

Answer Key: 1. hyperthyroidism 2. prosthesis 3. diarrhea 4. tachycardia 5. dysplasia 6. ultrasonography 7. metastasis 8. dialysis 9. tricuspid 10. transurethral 11. malignant 12. congenital 13. endocrine 14. antigen 15. ectopic pregnancy 16. subtotal

J.   Use the following terms to complete the sentences below:

transurethral	relapse	incision	analysis
prolapse	neoplastic	post partum	paralysis
neonatal	tachycardia	post mortem	anemia
remission	resection	ante partum	

1. Complete removal of Ms. Smith's stomach was necessary because of the presence of an adenocarcinoma. Dr. Nife performed the gastric _____.

2. After she had nine children, Ms. Gravida's uterine walls became weak, causing her uterus to fall and _____ through her vagina.

3. The autopsy or _____ examination of a dead body is an important step in determining the cause of death.

4. After Mr. Puffer's heart attack, doctors were concerned because he continued to have a persistent, rapid, abnormal heart rhythm. They prescribed drugs called antiarrhythmics to treat his _____.

5. The special ward in the hospital devoted to newborn babies is known as the _____ unit.

6. Ms. Rowe was pleased that she hadn't had symptoms of her malignant disease for the past six years. Her illness was in _____.

7. The operation to remove part of Mr. Jones' enlarged (hypertrophied) prostate gland involved placing a catheter through his urethra and removing pieces of the prostate through the tube. The surgery is called a _____ resection of the prostate gland (TURP). The prostate gland is located at the base of the bladder in males. See Figure 4–12.

8. Mr. M. Pathy was in a sad mood for several weeks after his wife had their first baby. He was experiencing a(an) _____ depression.

9. Ms. Smith's recent stroke left her with loss of muscle movement on the right side of her body, also called right-sided _____.

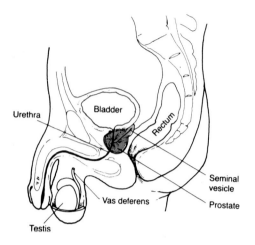

Urethra

Bladder

Rectum

Seminal
vesicle

Vas deferens

Prostate

Testis

FIGURE 4–12. Prostate gland.

10. Excessive bleeding or lack of iron in diet can lead to a decrease of hemoglobin in red blood cells, a condition known as iron-deficiency _____.

Answer Key: 1. resection   2. prolapse   3. post mortem   4. tachycardia
5. neonatal   6. remission   7. transurethral   8. post partum   9. paralysis   10. anemia

K. Underline the term that is spelled correctly and give the meaning of the term:

1. adnormal   abnormal   _____

2. bradycardia   bradicardia   _____

3. dysuria   disuria   _____

4. perriosteum   periosteum   _____

5. subcutaneous   subcutanous   _____

6. metastatis   metastasis   _____

7. parathyriod   parathyroid   _____

8. diarheea   diarrhea   _____

9. antebiotic   antibiotic   _____

10. incission   incision   _____

Answer Key: 1. abnormal—away from the rule, order of things   2. bradycardia
—slow heartbeat   3. dysuria—painful urination   4. periosteum—surrounding
the bone   5. subcutaneous—under the skin   6. metastasis—spreading of a
cancerous tumor to another location   7. parathyroid—glands that are located on
the backside of the thyroid gland   8. diarrhea—watery discharge from the
colon   9. antibiotic—substance produced by molds to fight against bacteria
10. incision—to cut into

V. REVIEW

PART A: PREFIXES

Write the meanings for the following prefixes, and please don't forget to check your answers!

1.	a-, an-	_____	11.	dys-	_____
2.	ab-	_____	12.	ec-	_____
3.	ad-	_____	13.	endo-	_____
4.	ana-	_____	14.	epi-	_____
5.	ante-	_____	15.	ex-, extra-	_____
6.	anti-	_____	16.	hyper-	_____
7.	bi-	_____	17.	hypo-	_____
8.	brady-	_____	18.	in-	_____
9.	con-	_____	19.	inter-	_____
10.	dia-	_____	20.	intra-	_____

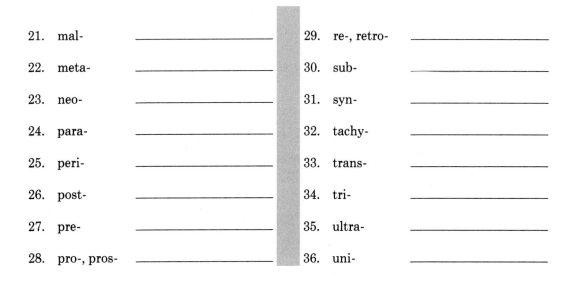

21. mal- _____
22. meta- _____
23. neo- _____
24. para- _____
25. peri- _____
26. post- _____
27. pre- _____
28. pro-, pros- _____

29. re-, retro- _____
30. sub- _____
31. syn- _____
32. tachy- _____
33. trans- _____
34. tri- _____
35. ultra- _____
36. uni- _____

PART B: COMBINING FORMS

Write the meaning of each combining form in the space provided.

1. abdomin/o _____
2. an/o _____
3. bi/o _____
4. cardi/o _____
5. carp/o _____
6. cis/o _____
7. cost/o _____
8. crani/o _____
9. cutane/o _____
10. dur/o _____
11. gen/o _____

12. glyc/o _____
13. hemat/o _____
14. later/o _____
15. nat/i _____
16. norm/o _____
17. oste/o _____
18. peritone/o _____
19. plas/o _____
20. ren/o _____
21. scapul/o _____
22. son/o _____

23. thyroid/o _____   27. uter/o _____

24. top/o _____   28. ven/o _____

25. troph/o _____   29. vertebr/o _____

26. urethr/o _____

PART C: SUFFIXES

Write the meanings for the following suffixes in the spaces indicated below.

1. -al _____   15. -ous _____

2. -ation _____   16. -partum _____

3. -cision _____   17. -plasm _____

4. -crine _____   18. -pnea _____

5. -emia _____   19. -rrhea _____

6. -gen _____   20. -scopy _____

7. -graphy _____   21. -section _____

8. -ia _____   22. -stasis _____

9. -ic _____   23. -tension _____

10. -ine _____   24. -thesis _____

11. -ism _____   25. -tic _____

12. -lysis _____   26. -um _____

13. -mortem _____   27. -uria _____

14. -oma _____   28. -y _____

PREFIXES

Answer Key: 1. no, not, without   2. away from   3. toward   4. up, apart
5. before, forward   6. against   7. two   8. slow   9. with, together
10. through, complete   11. bad, painful, difficult   12. out, outside
13. within, in, inner   14. above, upon   15. out, outside   16. excessive,
above   17. below, under   18. in, into   19. between   20. within
21. bad   22. beyond   23. new   24. near, along the side of   25. surrounding   26. after, behind   27. before   28. before, forward   29. back, behind   30. beneath, less than   31. with, together   32. fast   33. across,
through   34. three   35. beyond   36. one

COMBINING FORMS

Answer Key: 1. abdomen   2. anus   3. life   4. heart   5. wrist bones
6. to cut   7. ribs   8. skull   9. skin   10. dura mater   11. to produce
12. sugar   13. blood   14. side   15. birth   16. rule, order   17. bone
18. peritoneum   19. formation, growth   20. kidney   21. shoulder blade
(bone)   22. sound   23. thyroid gland   24. to put, place   25. development,
nourishment   26. urethra   27. uterus   28. vein   29. vertebra (backbone)

SUFFIXES

Answer Key: 1. pertaining to   2. process, condition   3. process of cutting
4. secretion   5. blood condition   6. to produce   7. process of recording
8. condition, process   9. pertaining to   10. pertaining to   11. condition,
process   12. loosening, breakdown, separation, destruction   13. death
14. tumor   15. pertaining to   16. birth   17. formation   18. breathing
19. flow, discharge   20. process of examining   21. incision   22. stop,
control   23. pressure   24. to put, place   25. pertaining to   26. structure   27. urine condition   28. process, condition

VI. PRONUNCIATION OF TERMS

Say each word out loud as you pronounce it, and then write its meaning in the space provided.

Term	*Pronunciation*	*Meaning*
abnormal	ab-**NOR**-mal	_____
adrenal glands	ad-**RE**-nal glanz	_____
analysis	ah-**NAL**-ih-sis	_____
anemia	ah-**NE**-me-ah	_____
ante mortem	**AN**-te **MOR**-tem	_____
ante partum	**AN**-te **PAR**-tum	_____
antenatal	**AN**-te **NA**-tal	_____
antibiotic	an-tih-bi-**OT**-ik	_____
antibodies	an-tih-**BOD**-eez	_____
antigen	**AN**-tih-jen	_____
apnea	**AP**-ne-ah	_____
atrophy	**AT**-ro-fe	_____
benign	Be-**NIN**	_____
bilateral	bi-**LAT**-er-al	_____
bradycardia	bra-de-**KAR**-de-ah	_____
congenital anomaly	kon-**JEN**-ih-tal ah-**NOM**-ah-le	_____
dialysis	di-**AL**-ih-sis	_____
diarrhea	di-ah-**RE**-ah	_____
dysplasia	dis-**PLA**-se-ah	_____

dyspnea	**DISP**-ne-ah _____
dysuria	dis-**U**-re-ah _____
ectopic pregnancy	ek-**TOP**-ik **PREG**-nan-se _____
endocrine glands	**EN**-do-krin glanz _____
endoscopy	en-**DOS**-ko-pe _____
epidural hematoma	ep-ih-**DUR**-al he-mah-**TO**-mah _____
excision	ek-**SIZH**-un _____
extrahepatic	eks-tra-heh-**PAT**-ik _____
hyperglycemia	hi-per-gli-**SE**-me-ah _____
hypertension	hi-per-**TEN**-shun _____
hyperthyroidism	hi-per-**THI**-royd-izm _____
hypertrophy	hi-**PER**-tro-fe _____
hypoglycemia	hi-po-gli-**SE**-me-ah _____
incision	in-**SIZH**-un _____
intervertebral	in-ter-**VER**-teh-bral _____
intrauterine	in-tra-**U**-ter-in _____
intravenous	in-trah-**VE**-nus _____
malignant	mah-**LIG**-nant _____
metacarpal	met-ah-**KAR**-pal _____
metastasis	meh-**TAS**-tah-sis _____
neonatal	ne-o-**NA**-tal _____
neoplastic	ne-o-**PLAS**-tik _____
paralysis	pah-**RAL**-ih-sis _____

parathyroid glands	par-ah-**THI**-royd glanz _____
perianal	per-e-**A**-nal _____
periosteum	per-e-**OS**-te-um _____
polyuria	pol-e-**UR**-e-ah _____
post mortem	post **MOR**-tem _____
post partum	post **PAR**-tum _____
precancerous	pre-**KAN**-ser-us _____
prolapse	pro-**LAPS** _____
prosthesis	pros-**THE**-sis _____
relapse	re-**LAPS** _____
remission	re-**MISH**-un _____
resection	re-**SEK**-shun _____
retroperitoneal	reh-tro-per-ih-to-**NE**-al _____
subcostal	sub-**KOS**-tal _____
subcutaneous	sub-ku-**TA**-ne-us _____
subdural hematoma	sub-**DUR**-al he-mah-**TO**-mah _____
subscapular	sub-**SKAP**-u-lar _____
subtotal	sub-**TO**-tal _____
syndrome	**SIN**-drom _____
tachycardia	tak-eh-**KAR**-de-ah _____
tachypnea	tak-ip-**NE**-ah _____
transabdominal	trans-ab-**DOM**-ih-nal _____
transurethral	trans-u-**RE**-thral _____

tricuspid valve	tri-**KUS**-pid valv	_____
ultrasonography	ul-trah-son-**OG**-rah-fe	_____
unilateral	u-nih-**LAT**-er-al	_____
urinalysis	u-rih-**NAL**-ih-sis	_____

CHAPTER 5

MEDICAL SPECIALISTS AND CASE REPORTS

CHAPTER OBJECTIVES

- To describe the training process of physicians
- To identify medical specialists and describe their specialties
- To identify combining forms used in terms that describe specialists
- To decipher medical terminology as written in case reports

I. INTRODUCTION

This chapter reviews many of the terms you have learned in previous chapters while adding others related to medical specialists. In Section II, the training of physicians is described and specialists are listed with their specialties. Section III uses combining forms, which are found in the terms describing specialists, with familiar suffixes to test your knowledge of terms. In Section IV, short case reports are presented to illustrate the use of the medical language in context. As you read these reports, you will be impressed with your ability to understand medical terminology!

II. MEDICAL SPECIALISTS

Doctors complete four years of medical school and, after passing National Medical Board Examinations, receive an M.D. (Medical Doctor) degree. They may then begin postgraduate training, the length of which is at least three years, and in some cases longer. This postgraduate training is known as *residency training*. Examples of residency programs are:

Anesthesiology	Administration of agents capable of bringing about a loss of sensation
Dermatology	Diagnosis and treatment of skin disorders
Emergency medicine	Care of patients that requires sudden and immediate action
Family medicine	Primary care of all members of the family on a continuing basis
Internal medicine	Diagnosis of disorders and treatment with drugs
Ophthalmology	Diagnosis and treatment of eye disorders
Pathology	Diagnosis of disease by analysis of cells and tissues
Pediatrics	Diagnosis and treatment of children's disorders
Psychiatry	Diagnosis and treatment of disorders of the mind
Radiology	Diagnosis of disease using x-rays
Surgery	Treatment by manual (hand) or operative methods

Examinations are administered after completion of each residency program to certify competency in that specialty area.

A physician may then choose to specialize further by doing *fellowship* training. Fellowships (two to five years) train doctors in *clinical* (patient care) and *research* (laboratory) skills. For example, an *internist* (specialist in internal medicine) may choose fellowship training in internal medical specialties such as neurology, nephrology, endocrinology, and oncology. A surgeon interested in further specialization may do fellowship training in thoracic surgery, neurosurgery, or plastic surgery. Upon completion of training and examinations, the doctor is then a recognized specialist in that specialty area.

Medical specialists and an explanation of their specialties are listed below:

Medical Specialist	*Specialty*
allergist	Treatment of hypersensitivity reactions
anesthesiologist	Administration of agents for loss of sensation
cardiologist	Treatment of heart disease
cardiovascular surgeon	Surgery on the heart and blood vessels
colorectal surgeon	Surgery on the colon and rectum
dermatologist	Treatment of skin disorders
endocrinologist	Treatment of endocrine gland disorders
gastroenterologist	Treatment of stomach and intestinal disorders
geriatrician	Treatment of diseases of old age
gynecologist	Surgery and treatment of the female reproductive system
hematologist	Treatment of blood disorders
infectious disease specialist	Treatment of diseases caused by microorganisms
nephrologist	Treatment of kidney diseases
neurologist	Treatment of nerve disorders
neurosurgeon	Surgery on the brain, spinal cord, and nerves
obstetrician	Treatment of pregnant women; delivery of babies
oncologist	Treatment of malignant tumors
ophthalmologist	Surgical and medical treatment of eye disorders
orthopedist	Surgical treatment of bones, muscles, and joints
otolaryngologist	Treatment of the ear, nose, and throat
pathologist	Diagnosis of disease by analysis of cells
pediatrician	Treatment of diseases of children
physical medicine and rehabilitation specialist	Treatment to restore function after illness
psychiatrist	Treatment of mental disorders
pulmonary specialist	Treatment of lung diseases
radiologist	Examination of x-rays to determine a diagnosis
radiotherapist	Treatment of disease with high-energy radiation
rheumatologist	Treatment of joint and muscle disorders
thoracic surgeon	Surgery on chest organs
urologist	Surgery on the urinary tract

III.   COMBINING FORMS AND VOCABULARY

The combining forms listed below are familiar because they are found in the terms describing medical specialists. A medical term is included to illustrate the use of the combining form. Write the meaning of the medical term in the space provided. You can always check your answers with the *Glossary* at the end of the book.

Combining Form	Meaning	Medical Term	Meaning
cardi/o	heart	cardiomegaly	_____
col/o	colon	colostomy	_____
dermat/o	skin	dermatitis	_____
endocrin/o	endocrine glands	endocrinology	_____
enter/o	intestines	enteritis	_____
esthesi/o	sensation	anesthesiology	_____
gastr/o	stomach	gastroscopy	_____
ger/o	old age	geriatrics	_____
gynec/o	woman, female	gynecology	_____
hemat/o	blood	hematoma	_____
iatr/o	treatment	iatrogenic	_____

IATR/O means treatment by a physician or with medicines. An iatrogenic illness is *produced* (-genic) unexpectedly by a treatment.

Combining Form	Meaning	Medical Term	Meaning
laryng/o	voice box	laryngeal	_____
nephr/o	kidney	nephrostomy	_____
neur/o	nerve	neuralgia	_____
obstetr/o	midwife	obstetric	_____

onc/o	tumor	oncogenic _____ Oncogenic viruses produce tumors.
ophthalm/o	eye	ophthalmologist _____
opt/o	eye	optometrist _____ An optometrist examines (METR means "measure") eyes and prescribes glasses but cannot treat eye diseases.
		optician _____ Opticians grind lenses and fit glasses but do not examine eyes, prescribe glasses, or treat eye diseases.
orth/o	straight	orthopedist _____ PED/O comes from the Greek, *paidos,* meaning "child." Orthopedists in the past were concerned with straightening bone deformities in children.
ot/o	ear	otitis _____
path/o	disease	pathology _____
ped/o	child	pediatrics _____
psych/o	mind	psychosis _____
pulmon/o	lung	pulmonary _____
radi/o	x-rays	radiotherapy _____
rect/o	rectum	rectocele _____ -CELE means "a hernia or protrusion." The walls of the rectum weaken and bulge forward toward the vagina. See Figure 5–1.
rheumat/o	flow, fluid	rheumatology _____ Joints can fill with fluid when diseased, hence RHEUMAT/O indicates a problem with a swollen joint. Rheumatoid arthritis is a chronic inflammatory dis-

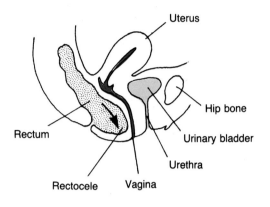

FIGURE 5–1. Rectocele.

		ease of joints and connective tissues which leads to deformation of joints. See Figure 5–2.
rhin/o	nose	rhinorrhea _____
thorac/o	chest	thoracotomy _____
ur/o	urinary tract	urology _____
vascul/o	blood vessels	vasculitis _____

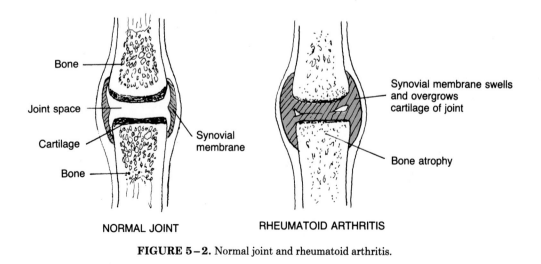

FIGURE 5–2. Normal joint and rheumatoid arthritis.

IV. CASE REPORTS

Here are short reports related to medical specialties. Many terms are familiar, others are explained in the *Glossary*. Write the meaning of the underlined term in the space provided.

CASE 1: CARDIOLOGY

Mr. Rose was admitted to the Cardiac Care Unit (CCU) following a severe *myocardial infarction*. He had suffered from *angina* (due to *ischemia*), and *hypertension* for some time previously. He is being treated with *antiarrhythmic* drugs, *diuretics,* and *anticoagulants.* If his recovery proceeds as expected, he will be discharged in three weeks.

angina _____

antiarrhythmic _____

anticoagulant _____

diuretic _____

hypertension _____

ischemia _____

myocardial infarction _____

CASE 2: GYNECOLOGY

Ms. Sessions has been complaining of *dysmenorrhea* and *menorrhagia* for several months. She is also *anemic.* Because of the presence of large *fibroids,* as seen on a pelvic *ultrasound* exam (*sonogram*), *hysterectomy* is recommended.

anemic _____

dysmenorrhea _____

fibroids _____

hysterectomy _____

menorrhagia _____

sonogram _____

ultrasound _____

CASE 3: ONCOLOGY

The patient is a 26-year-old female with a previous diagnosis of *mediastinal* and *intra-abdominal Hodgkin's disease.* She is admitted to the hospital for *lymphangiography* and *percutaneous* liver *biopsy* after discovery of possible recurrence of tumor.

Following the assessment of her *platelet* count, a percutaneous liver biopsy was performed and showed normal *hepatic* tissue. The *lymphangiogram* was normal as well. The patient was later scheduled for *peritoneoscopy.*

biopsy _____

hepatic _____

Hodgkin's disease _____

intra-abdominal _____

lymphangiogram _____

lymphangiography _____

mediastinal _____

percutaneous _____

peritoneoscopy _____

platelet _____

CASE 4: UROLOGY

Polly Smith has a history of lower back pain associated with *hematuria* and *dysuria.* She has an appointment at the hospital for investigation of her symptoms.

Tests include an *intravenous pyelogram* (IVP) and *cystoscopy*.

The findings of these tests confirm the diagnosis of *renal calculus. Lithotripsy* is recommended and *prognosis* is favorable.

calculus _____

cystoscopy _____

dysuria _____

hematuria _____

intravenous pyelogram (IVP) _____

lithotripsy _____

prognosis _____

renal _____

CASE 5: GASTROENTEROLOGY

Mr. Pepper suffers from *dyspepsia* and sharp *abdominal* pain. A recent episode of *hematemesis* has left him very weak and *anemic*.

Gastroscopy and *barium enema* revealed the presence of a large *ulcer*. He will be admitted to the hospital and scheduled for a partial *gastrectomy*.

abdominal _____

anemic _____

barium enema _____

dyspepsia _____

gastrectomy _____

gastroscopy _____

hematemesis _____

ulcer _____

CASE 6: RADIOLOGY

Examination: *Thoracic cavity*

PA (*posterior-anterior*) and *lateral* chest. There is a patchy *infiltrate* in the right lower *lobe* seen best in the lateral view. The heart and *mediastinal* structures are normal. No evidence of *pleural effusion*.

Impression: Right lower lobe *pneumonia*

anterior _____

infiltrate _____

lateral _____

lobe _____

mediastinal _____

pleural effusion _____

pneumonia _____

posterior _____

thoracic cavity _____

CASE 7: ORTHOPEDICS

A 20-year-old male patient was admitted to the hospital following a motor-cycle accident. In the accident he sustained *fractures* of the right *tibia*, right *femur*, and *pelvis* and *intra-abdominal* injuries.

Two pins were placed through the lower and upper end of the tibia and a cast was applied. Two days later he was taken to surgery and internal *fixation* of the right femur was performed.

femur _____

fixation _____

fracture _____

intra-abdominal _____

pelvis _____

tibia _____

CASE 8: NEPHROLOGY

A 52-year-old man with *chronic renal failure* secondary to long-standing *hypertension* has been maintained on *hemodialysis* for the past 18 months. For the past three weeks during the dialysis sessions he has become moderately *hypotensive,* with symptoms of dizziness. Consequently, we have decided to withhold his *antihypertensive* medications prior to dialysis.

antihypertensive _____

chronic _____

hemodialysis _____

hypertension _____

hypotensive _____

renal failure _____

CASE 9: ENDOCRINOLOGY

A 36-year-old woman known to have *insulin*-dependent *diabetes mellitus* was brought to the emergency room after being found collapsed in her home. She had experienced three days of extreme weakness, *polyuria,* and *polydipsia.* It was discovered that a few days prior to her admission she had discontinued her insulin in a suicide attempt.

diabetes mellitus _____

insulin _____

polydipsia _____

polyuria _____

CASE 10: NEUROLOGY

Mary Ann Rose is admitted with severe, throbbing *unilateral frontal cephalgia* that has lasted for two days. Light makes her cringe and she complains of *nausea.* Before the onset of these symptoms, she saw zigzag lines for about 20 minutes. Diagnosis is *acute migraine* with *aura*. A *vasoconstrictor* is prescribed, and Ms. Rose's condition is improving. (Migraine headaches are thought to be caused by sudden *dilation* of blood vessels.)

acute _____

aura _____

cephalgia _____

dilation _____

frontal _____

migraine _____

nausea _____

unilateral _____

vasoconstrictor _____

V. EXERCISES

These exercises test your understanding of the terms in Sections II and III. Don't forget to check your responses with the answers directly following each exercise.

A. *Match the following residency programs with their descriptions that follow:*

internal medicine	pediatrics	psychiatry
radiology	surgery	family medicine
anesthesiology	emergency medicine	pathology
dermatology	ophthalmology	

1. Treatment by operation or manual (hand) methods: _____

2. Diagnosis of disorders and treatment with drugs: _____

3. Diagnosis and treatment of disorders of the mind: _____

4. Care of family members on a continuing basis: _____

5. Diagnosis and treatment of skin disorders: _____

6. Diagnosis and treatment of eye disorders: _____

7. Diagnosis of disease using x-rays: _____

8. Diagnosis and treatment of children's disorders: _____

9. Care of patients that requires immediate action: _____

10. Administration of agents that cause loss of sensation: _____

11. Diagnosis of disease by examining cells and tissues: _____

Answer Key: 1. surgery   2. internal medicine   3. psychiatry   4. family medicine   5. dermatology   6. ophthalmology   7. radiology   8. pediatrics   9. emergency medicine   10. anesthesiology   11. pathology

B. *Name the doctor who treats the following problems (first letters are given):*

1. Kidney diseases   N _____

2. Tumors   O _____

3. Broken bones   O _____

4. Female diseases   G _____

5. Eye disorders   O _____

6. Heart disorders   C _____

7. Nerve disorders   N _____

8. Lung disorders   P _____

9. Mental disorders   P _____

10. Stomach and intestinal disorders   G _____

Answer Key: 1. nephrologist   2. oncologist   3. orthopedist   4. gynecologist   5. ophthalmologist   6. cardiologist (internist) or cardiovascular surgeon (surgeon)   7. neurologist   8. pulmonary specialist   9. psychiatrist   10. gastroenterologist

C. *Match the following medical specialists in Column I with their specialties in Column II:*

Column I		Column II
1. urologist	_____	A. Operates on the large intestine
		B. Treats blood disorders
2. thoracic surgeon	_____	C. Treats thyroid and pituitary gland disorders
		D. Delivers babies
3. radiotherapist	_____	E. Treats children and their disorders
		F. Operates on the urinary tract
4. colorectal surgeon	_____	G. Treats disorders of the skin
		H. Treats diseases by using high-energy radiation
5. endocrinologist	_____	I. Operates on the chest
		J. Examines x-rays to diagnose disease
6. obstetrician	_____	
7. radiologist	_____	
8. pediatrican	_____	
9. hematologist	_____	
10. dermatologist	_____	

Answer Key: 1. F   2. I   3. H   4. A   5. C   6. D   7. J   8. E   9. B   10. G

D. *Complete the sentences that follow using the terms listed below:*

clinical	orthopedist	optometrist	infectious disease specialist
pathologist	optician	research	geriatrician
ophthalmologist	oncologist	surgeon	

1. A physician who diagnoses and treats diseases that are caused by microorganisms is

   known as a(an) _____.

2. A doctor who does bone surgery is called a(an) _____.

3. A doctor who takes care of patients does _____ medicine.

4. A person who grinds lenses and fills prescriptions for eye glasses is called a(an)

    _____.

5. A doctor who reads biopsy samples and performs autopsies is called a(an)

    _____.

6. A doctor who treats cancerous tumors is called a(an) _____.

7. A person who can examine eyes and prescribe eye glasses but cannot treat eye disorders is

    called a(an) _____.

8. A doctor who operates on patients is called a(an) _____.

9. A doctor who does experiments with test tubes and laboratory equipment is interested in

    _____ medicine.

10. A doctor who specializes in treatment of disorders of the eye is called a(an)

    _____.

11. A doctor who specializes in the treatment of older people is called a(an)

    _____.

Answer Key: 1. infectious disease specialist   2. orthopedist   3. clinical
4. optician   5. pathologist   6. oncologist   7. optometrist   8. surgeon
9. research   10. ophthalmologist   11. geriatrician

E. *Which medical specialist would you consult for the following medical conditions? The first letter of the specialist is given.*

1. Arthritis   R _____

2. Otitis media   O _____

3. Anemia   H _____

4. Urinary bladder displacement   U _____

5. Chronic bronchitis   P _____

6. Cerebrovascular accident   N _____

7. Breast cancer   O _____

8. Hole in the wall of the heart   C _____

9. Dislocated shoulder bone   O _____

10. Thyroid gland enlargement   E _____

11. Kidney disease   N _____

12. Acne (skin disorder)   D _____

13. Hay fever (hypersensitivity reaction)   A _____

14. Viral and bacterial diseases   I _____

Answer Key: 1. rheumatologist   2. otolaryngologist   3. hematologist
4. urologist   5. pulmonary specialist   6. neurologist   7. oncologist
8. cardiovascular surgeon   9. orthopedist   10. endocrinologist   11. nephrologist   12. dermatologist   13. allergist   14. infectious disease specialist

F. *Give meanings for the following medical terms:*

1. neuralgia _____

2. pathology _____

3. cardiomegaly _____

4. nephrostomy _____

5. thoracotomy _____

6. laryngeal _____

7. otitis _____

8. colostomy _____

9. pulmonary _____

10. iatrogenic _____

11. gastroscopy _____

12. radiotherapy _____

13. anesthesiology _____

14. enteritis _____

Answer Key: 1. nerve pain   2. study of disease   3. enlargement of the heart   4. opening from the kidney to the outside of the body   5. incision of the chest   6. pertaining to the voice box   7. inflammation of the ear   8. opening of the colon to the outside of the body   9. pertaining to the lungs   10. pertaining to an abnormal condition that has been produced by treatment   11. process of visual examination of the stomach   12. treatment of disease using high-energy radiation   13. study of loss of sensation or feeling   14. inflammation of the intestines (usually small intestine)

G. *Use the following combining forms and suffixes to make the medical terms called for:*

Combining Forms		Suffixes	
laryng/o	nephr/o	-itis	-scopy
neur/o	ophthalm/o	-ectomy	-osis
onc/o	thorac/o	-tomy	-logy
col/o	ot/o	-algia	-therapy
psych/o	path/o	-genic	-stomy

1. Inflammation of the ear: _____

2. Removal of a nerve: _____

3. Incision of the chest: _____

4. Study of tumors: _____

5. Pertaining to producing disease: _____

6. Inflammation of the voice box: _____

7. Opening of the large intestine to the outside of the body: _____

8. Visual examination of the eye: _____

9. Abnormal condition of the mind: _____

10. Inflammation of the kidney: _____

11. Removal of the large intestine: _____

12. Pain in the ear: _____

13. Treatment of the mind: _____

14. Pertaining to producing tumors: _____

Answer Key: 1. otitis   2. neurectomy   3. thoracotomy   4. oncology
5. pathogenic   6. laryngitis   7. colostomy   8. ophthalmoscopy   9. psychosis   10. nephritis   11. colectomy   12. otalgia   13. psychotherapy
14. oncogenic

H. Circle the term that is spelled correctly and give the meaning of the term:

1. pschiatrist   psychiatrist   _____

2. neuralgia   nueralgia   _____

3. cardiomegaly   cardiomeagaly   _____

4. rheumatologist   rhumatologist   _____

5. opthalmascope   ophthalmoscope   _____

6. laryngitis   laringitis   _____

7. onkologist   oncologist   _____

8. anesthiology   anesthesiology   _____

9. pediatrian   pediatrician   _____

10. gastroenteroitis   gastroenteritis   _____

11. gynecology   gynocology   _____

12. rectosele   rectocele   _____

Answer Key: 1. psychiatrist — one who treats disorders of the mind   2. neuralgia — nerve pain   3. cardiomegaly — enlargement of the heart   4. rheumatologist — one who treats diseases of joints   5. ophthalmoscope — instrument to examine the eye   6. laryngitis — inflammation of the voice box   7. oncologist — one who specializes in the study of tumors   8. anesthesiology — study of producing loss of sensation   9. pediatrician — one who treats children   10. gastroenteritis — inflammation of the stomach and intestines   11. gynecology — study of female disorders   12. rectocele — hernia of the rectum

VI. REVIEW

Test your understanding of the combining forms and suffixes in this chapter by completing the following REVIEW exercise:

COMBINING FORMS

Combining Form	Meaning		Combining Form	Meaning
1. cardi/o	_____		8. ger/o	_____
2. col/o	_____		9. gynec/o	_____
3. dermat/o	_____		10. hemat/o	_____
4. endocrin/o	_____		11. iatr/o	_____
5. enter/o	_____		12. laryng/o	_____
6. esthesi/o	_____		13. nephr/o	_____
7. gastr/o	_____		14. neur/o	_____

Combining Form	Meaning		Combining Form	Meaning
15. obstetr/o	_____		24. pulmon/o	_____
16. onc/o	_____		25. radi/o	_____
17. ophthalm/o	_____		26. rect/o	_____
18. opt/o	_____		27. rheumat/o	_____
19. orth/o	_____		28. rhin/o	_____
20. ot/o	_____		29. thorac/o	_____
21. path/o	_____		30. ur/o	_____
22. ped/o	_____		31. vascul/o	_____
23. psych/o	_____			

SUFFIXES

Suffix	Meaning		Suffix	Meaning
1. -algia	_____		9. -megaly	_____
2. -ary	_____		10. -oma	_____
3. -cele	_____		11. -osis	_____
4. -eal	_____		12. -rrhea	_____
5. -genic	_____		13. -scopy	_____
6. -ist	_____		14. -stomy	_____
7. -itis	_____		15. -therapy	_____
8. -logy	_____		16. -tomy	_____

COMBINING FORMS

Answer Key: 1. heart 2. colon 3. skin 4. endocrine glands 5. intestines 6. sensation 7. stomach 8. old age 9. woman 10. blood 11. treatment 12. voice box 13. kidney 14. nerve 15. midwife 16. tumor 17. eye 18. eye 19. straight 20. ear 21. disease 22. child 23. mind 24. lung 25. x-rays 26. rectum 27. flow, fluid 28. nose 29. chest 30. urinary tract 31. blood vessels

SUFFIXES

Answer Key: 1. pain 2. pertaining to 3. hernia, protrusion 4. pertaining to 5. pertaining to producing 6. specialist 7. inflammation 8. study of 9. enlargement 10. mass, tumor 11. abnormal condition 12. flow 13. process of visual examination 14. opening 15. treatment 16. incision

VII. PRONUNCIATION OF TERMS

Say each word out loud as you pronounce it, and then write its meaning in the space provided.

Term	Pronunciation	Meaning
anesthesiology	an-es-the-ze-**OL**-o-je	_____
cardiologist	kar-de-**OL**-o-jist	_____
cardiovascular surgeon	kar-de-o-**VAS**-ku-lar **SUR**-jin	_____
clinical	**KLIN**-eh-kal	_____
colorectal surgeon	ko-lo-**REK**-tal **SUR**-jin	_____
colostomy	ko-**LOS**-to-me	_____
dermatologist	der-mah-**TOL**-o-jist	_____
dermatology	der-mah-**TOL**-o-je	_____

emergency medicine	e-**MER**-jen-se **MED**-ih-sin _____
endocrinologist	en-do-krih-**NOL**-o-jist _____
enteritis	en-teh-**RI**-tis _____
family medicine	**FAM**-ih-le **MED**-ih-sin _____
gastroenterologist	gas-tro-en-ter-**OL**-o-jist _____
gastroscopy	gas-**TROS**-ko-pe _____
geriatric	jer-e-**AH**-trik _____
geriatrician	jer-e-ah-**TRISH**-shun _____
gynecologist	gi-neh-**KOL**-o-jist _____
gynecology	gi-neh-**KOL**-o-je _____
hematologist	he-mah-**TOL**-o-jist _____
hematoma	he-mah-**TO**-mah _____
iatrogenic	i-ah-tro-**JEN**-ik _____
infectious disease	in-**FEK**-shus dih-**ZEZ** _____
internal medicine	in-**TER**-nal **MED**-ih-sin _____
laryngitis	lah-rin-**JI**-tis _____
nephrologist	neh-**FROL**-o-jist _____
nephrostomy	neh-**FROS**-to-me _____
neuralgia	nu-**RAL**-je-ah _____
neurologist	nu-**ROL**-o-jist _____
neurosurgeon	nu-ro-**SUR**-jin _____
obstetrician	ob-steh-**TRISH**-un _____
obstetrics	ob-**STET**-riks _____

oncogenic	ong-ko-**JEN**-ik
oncologist	ong-**KOL**-o-jist
ophthalmologist	of-thal-**MOL**-o-jist
ophthalmology	of-thal-**MOL**-o-je
optician	op-**TISH**-un
optometrist	op-**TOM**-eh-trist
orthopedist	orth-o-**PE**-dist
otitis	o-**TI**-tis
otolaryngologist	o-to-lar-in-**GOL**-o-jist
pathologist	pah-**THOL**-o-jist
pathology	pah-**THOL**-o-je
pediatric	pe-de-**AT**-rik
pediatrician	pe-de-ah-**TRISH**-un
psychiatrist	si-**KI**-ah-trist
psychosis	si-**KO**-sis
pulmonary specialist	**PUL**-mo-ner-e **SPESH**-ah-list
radiologist	ra-de-**OL**-o-jist
radiotherapist	ra-de-o-**THER**-ah-pist
radiotherapy	ra-de-o-**THER**-ah-pe
rectocele	**REK**-to-sel
research	**RE**-surch
rheumatologist	ru-mah-**TOL**-o-jist
rheumatology	ru-mah-**TOL**-o-je

rhinorrhea	ri-no-**RE**-ah ————————————
surgery	**SIR**-jer-e ————————————
thoracic surgeon	tho-**RAS**-ik **SUR**-jin ————————————
thoracotomy	tho-rah-**KOT**-o-me ————————————
urologist	u-**ROL**-o-jist ————————————
vasculitis	vas-ku-**LI**-tis ————————————

APPENDIX I

BODY SYSTEMS

This appendix contains diagrams of the ten body systems. Major organs and structures are labeled for your reference, and definitions for these parts of the body are listed in the *Glossary of Medical Terms* on page 182. The combining forms used to describe parts of the body are found in the *Glossary of Word Parts* on page 208. This information will help you analyze medical terms as you work through the text. You will also find it useful as a reference for your work in the medical field.

The body systems are presented in alphabetical order as follows:

    I.   Circulatory System
   II.   Digestive System
  III.   Endocrine System
  IV.   Female Reproductive System
   V.   Male Reproductive System
  VI.   Musculoskeletal System
 VII.   Nervous System
VIII.   Respiratory System
  IX.   Skin and Sense Organs
   X.   Urinary System

I. CIRCULATORY SYSTEM

Circulation of Blood

Lung capillaries

Pulmonary
circulation

Left
atrium

aorta

heart

Right
atrium

Left
ventricle

Right
ventricle

arteries

veins

Systemic
circulation

venules

arterioles

tissue capillaries

Colored vessels contain blood that is rich in oxygen. Arrows show the path of blood flow from the tissue capillaries through venules and veins toward the heart, to the lung capillaries, back to the heart, out the aorta to the arteries and arterioles, and then to the tissue capillaries.

I. CIRCULATORY SYSTEM *(Continued)*

Circulation of Lymph

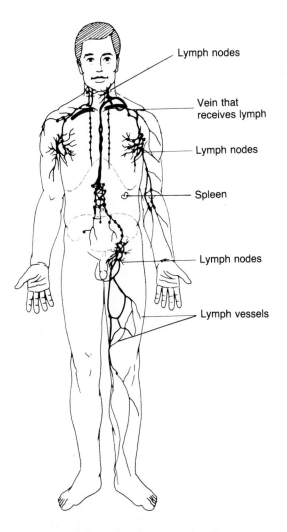

Lymph nodes

Vein that
receives lymph

Lymph nodes

Spleen

Lymph nodes

Lymph vessels

Lymph originates in the tissue spaces around cells, travels in lymph vessels and through lymph nodes to a large vein in the neck where it enters the bloodstream. Lymph contains white blood cells (lymphocytes) that help the body fight disease. The spleen produces lymphocytes and disposes of dying blood cells.

II. DIGESTIVE SYSTEM

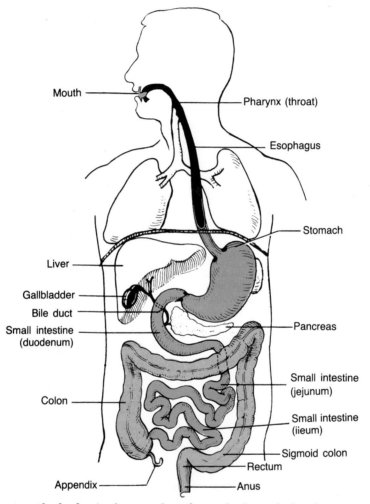

Food enters the body via the mouth and travels through the pharynx, esophagus, and stomach to the small intestine. The liver, gallbladder, and pancreas make and store chemicals that aid in the digestion of foods. Digested (broken down) food is absorbed into the bloodstream through the walls of the small intestine. Any food that cannot be absorbed continues into the colon (large intestine) and leaves the body through the rectum and anus.

III.   ENDOCRINE SYSTEM

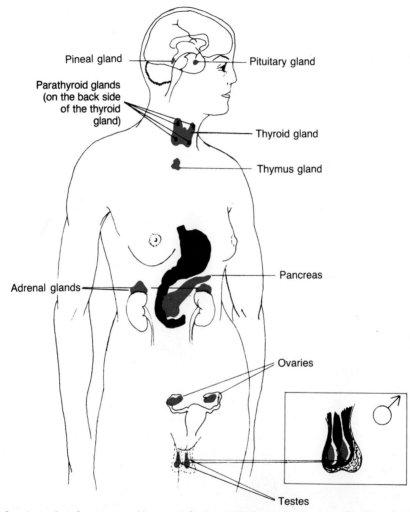

Pineal gland

Pituitary gland

Parathyroid glands
(on the back side
of the thyroid
gland)

Thyroid gland

Thymus gland

Pancreas

Adrenal glands

Ovaries

Testes

Endocrine glands secrete (form and give off) hormones into the bloodstream. The hormones travel throughout the body and affect organs (including other endocrine glands) to control their actions.

IV. FEMALE REPRODUCTIVE SYSTEM

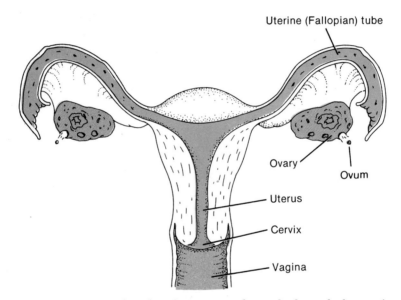

An egg cell (ovum) is produced in the ovary and travels through the uterine (fallopian) tube. If a sperm cell is present and fertilization (the union of the egg and sperm cell) takes place, the resulting cell (embryo) may implant in the lining of the uterus. The embryo (later called the fetus) develops in the uterus for nine months and is delivered from the body through the cervix and vagina.

V. MALE REPRODUCTIVE SYSTEM

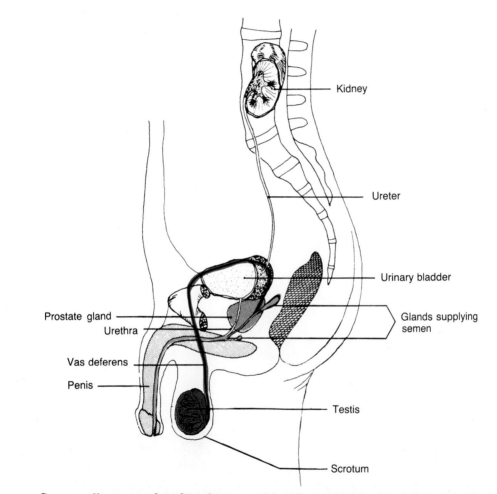

Kidney

Ureter

Urinary bladder

Glands supplying
semen

Prostate gland

Urethra

Vas deferens

Penis

Testis

Scrotum

Sperm cells are produced in the testes (singular: testis) and travel up into the body, through the vas deferens, and around the urinary bladder. The vas deferens unites with the urethra, which opens to the outside of the body through the penis. The prostate and the other glands near the urethra produce a fluid (semen) that leaves the body with sperm cells.

VI. MUSCULOSKELETAL SYSTEM

Bones: Anterior View

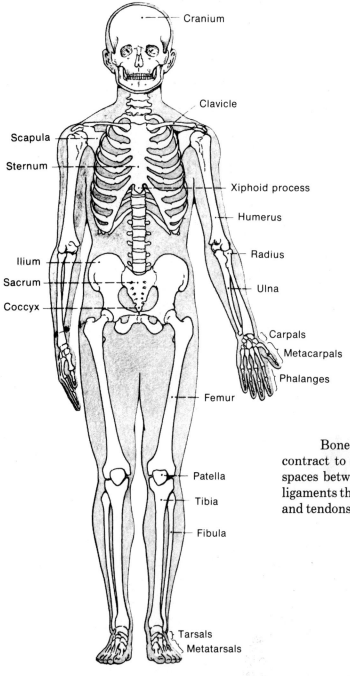

Cranium

Clavicle

Scapula

Sternum

Xiphoid process

Humerus

Radius

Ilium

Sacrum

Ulna

Coccyx

Carpals

Metacarpals

Phalanges

Femur

Patella

Tibia

Fibula

Tarsals

Metatarsals

Bones are connected to muscles that contract to move the body. Joints are the spaces between bones. Near the joints are ligaments that connect bones to other bones and tendons that connect bones to muscles.

VI. MUSCULOSKELETAL SYSTEM *(Continued)*

Bones: Posterior View

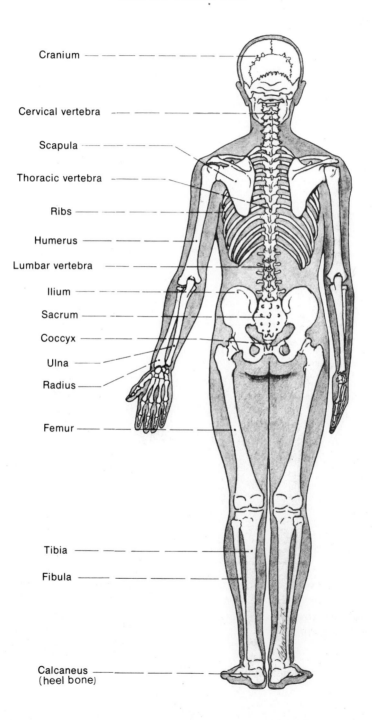

Cranium

Cervical vertebra

Scapula

Thoracic vertebra

Ribs

Humerus

Lumbar vertebra

Ilium

Sacrum

Coccyx

Ulna

Radius

Femur

Tibia

Fibula

Calcaneus
(heel bone)

VII. NERVOUS SYSTEM

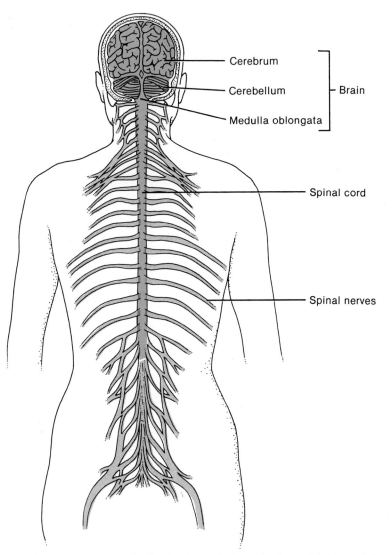

Cerebrum

Cerebellum

Medulla oblongata

Brain

Spinal cord

Spinal nerves

The central nervous system is the brain and the spinal cord. The peripheral nervous system includes the nerves that carry messages to and from the brain and spinal cord. Spinal nerves carry messages to and from the spinal cord, and the cranial nerves (not pictured) carry messages to and from the brain.

VIII. RESPIRATORY SYSTEM

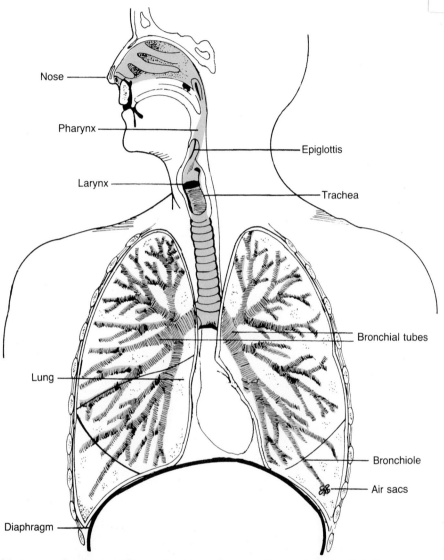

Air enters the nose and travels to the pharynx (throat). From the pharynx, air passes the epiglottis and larynx (voice box) into the trachea (windpipe). The trachea splits into two tubes, the bronchial tubes, that carry air into the lungs. The bronchial tubes divide into smaller tubes called bronchioles that end in small air sacs. The thin air sacs allow oxygen to pass through them into tiny capillaries containing red blood cells. The red blood cells transport the oxygen to all parts of the body.

In a similar manner, gaseous waste (carbon dioxide) leaves the blood to enter air sacs and then travels out of the body through bronchioles, bronchial tubes, trachea, larynx, pharynx, and the nose.

IX. SKIN AND SENSE ORGANS

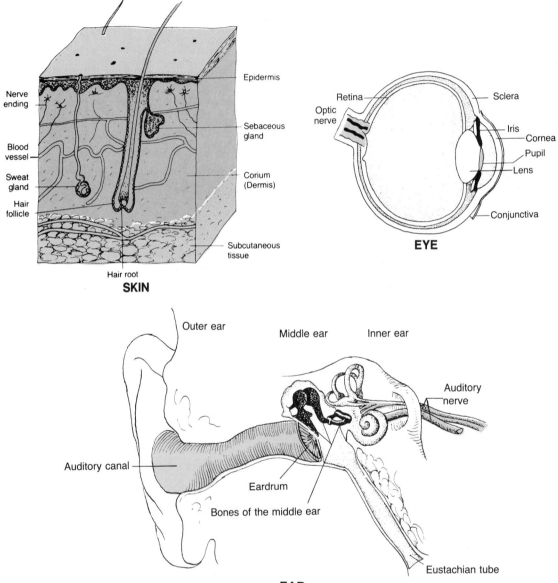

SKIN

Epidermis

Nerve ending

Blood vessel

Sweat gland

Hair follicle

Sebaceous gland

Corium (Dermis)

Subcutaneous tissue

Hair root

EYE

Retina

Optic nerve

Sclera

Iris

Cornea

Pupil

Lens

Conjunctiva

EAR

Outer ear

Middle ear

Inner ear

Auditory nerve

Auditory canal

Eardrum

Bones of the middle ear

Eustachian tube

The skin and sense organs receive messages (touch sensations, light waves, sound waves) from the environment and send them to the brain via nerves. These messages are interpreted in the brain, making sight, hearing, and perception of the environment possible.

X. URINARY SYSTEM

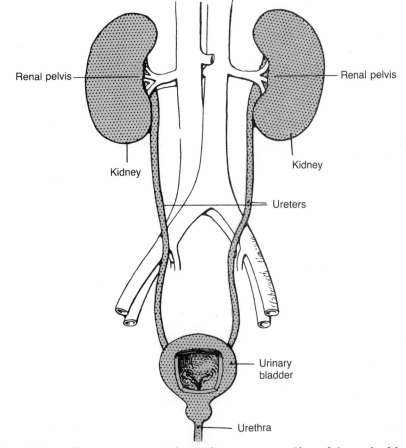

Renal pelvis — Kidney — Ureters — Urinary bladder — Urethra — Renal pelvis — Kidney

Urine is formed as waste materials, such as urea, are filtered from the blood into the tubules of the kidney. Urine passes from the tubules into the central collecting section of the kidney, the renal pelvis. Each renal pelvis leads directly to a ureter, which takes the urine to the urinary bladder. The bladder releases urine to the urethra and urine leaves the body.

APPENDIX II

DIAGNOSTIC TESTS AND PROCEDURES

Radiology, Ultrasound, and Imaging Procedures

In many of the following procedures a *dye* or *contrast* substance (medium) is introduced into or around a body part so that the part can be viewed while x-rays are taken. The contrast substance (often containing barium or iodine) appears dense on the x-ray and outlines the body part that it fills.

The suffix -GRAPHY, meaning "process of recording," is used in many terms describing imaging procedures. The suffix -GRAM, meaning "record," is also used and describes the actual image that is produced by the procedure.

Pronunciation of each term is given with its meaning. The syllable that gets the accent is in **CAPITAL LETTERS**.

ANGIOGRAPHY (an-je-OG-rah-fe) or ANGIOGRAM (AN-je-o-gram):   X-ray recording of blood vessels. Dye is injected into blood vessels (veins and arteries), and x-ray pictures are taken of the vessels. In *cerebral angiography,* x-ray pictures are taken of blood vessels in the brain. Angiography is used to detect abnormalities in blood vessels, such as blockage, malformation, and arteriosclerosis. Angiography is performed most frequently to view arteries and is often used interchangeably with arteriography.

ARTERIOGRAPHY (ar-ter-e-OG-rah-fe) or ARTERIOGRAM (ar-TER-e-o-gram):   X-ray recording of arteries after the introduction of dye into an artery. *Coronary arteriography* is the visualization of the arteries that bring blood to the heart muscle.

BARIUM ENEMA (BAH-re-um EN-eh-mah):   A liquid contrast substance called barium is injected through a plastic tube into the rectum and large intestine (colon). X-ray pictures of the colon are then taken. If tumor is present in the colon, it may appear as an obstruction or irregularity. This test is also called a *lower gastrointestinal (GI) exam.*

BARIUM SWALLOW (BAH-re-um SWAH-lo):   Barium sulfate is swallowed and x-ray pictures are taken of the esophagus, stomach, and small intestine. This test is also known as an *upper gastrointestinal (UGI) exam.* In a *small bowel follow-through,* pictures are taken at increasing time intervals to follow the progress of barium through the small intestine. Identification of obstructions or ulcers is possible.

BRONCHOGRAPHY (brong-KOG-rah-fe) or BRONCHOGRAM (BRONG-ko-gram):   X-ray recording of the bronchial tubes after contrast material (iodized oil) is instilled into the airways through a thin tube that is passed down through the trachea (windpipe). This procedure is used to investigate abnormalities of the bronchial tubes.

CARDIAC CATHETERIZATION (KAR-de-ak cath-eh-ter-i-ZA-shun):   A catheter (tube) is passed via a vein or artery into the chambers of the heart. This procedure may be used to measure the flow of blood out of the heart and the pressures and oxygen content in the heart chambers or to introduce a dye into the heart chambers so that x-ray pictures can be taken to show the structure of the heart.

CT SCAN, CAT SCAN: Also known as *computerized axial tomography,* this is a method of taking x-ray pictures to show the body in slices or cross-sections. Dye may be used (injected into the bloodstream) as contrast to highlight structures such as the liver, brain, or blood vessels, and barium may be swallowed to outline the gastrointestinal organs. X-ray pictures, taken as the x-ray tube rotates around the body, are processed by a computer to show images corresponding to a slice of body tissue. CT scans are taken of any area of the body but are most often used to visualize the brain, abdomen, and chest.

CEREBRAL ANGIOGRAPHY (seh-RE-bral an-je-OG-rah-fe): See ANGIOG:

CHOLANGIOGRAPHY (kol-an-je-OG-rah-fe) or CHOLANGIOGRAM (kol o-gram): X-ray recording of bile ducts. Dye is given by intravenous injection (*I.V. .... giogram*) and collects in the gallbladder and bile ducts or is directly inserted by a tube through the mouth into the bile ducts (*T-tube cholangiogram*). X-rays are taken of bile ducts (tubes that carry bile from the liver and gallbladder to the small intestine) to identify obstructions due to tumor or stones.

CHOLECYSTOGRAPHY (ko-le-sis-TOG-rah-fe) or CHOLECYSTOGRAM (ko-le-SIS-to-gram): X-ray recording of the gallbladder after intravenous or oral administration of contrast material. The test demonstrates the ability of the liver to clear the contrast material from the blood and excrete it in the bile; the ability of the gallbladder to fill and empty; and the presence of bile duct obstructions, such as gallstones, tumors, or other abnormalities. Also called a *gallbladder series*.

CORONARY ARTERIOGRAPHY (KOR-on-ar-e ar-ter-e-OG-rah-fe): See ARTERI-OGRAPHY.

CYSTOGRAPHY (sis-TOG-rah-fe) or CYSTOGRAM (SIS-to-gram): X-ray recording of the urinary bladder. Dye is injected through the urethra into the urinary bladder, and x-rays are taken of the bladder.

DIGITAL SUBTRACTION ANGIOGRAPHY (DIJ-i-tal sub-TRAK-shun an-je-OG-rah-fe): A special x-ray technique for viewing blood vessels. Images are taken first without injection of dye and then again after dye is injected into vessels. The first picture is then subtracted from the second so that the final image (sharp and precise) shows only the dye-filled blood vessels minus the surrounding tissue.

ECHOCARDIOGRAPHY (eh-ko-kar-de-OG-rah-fe) or ECHOCARDIOGRAM (eh-ko-KAR-de-o-gram): Images of the heart are produced by introducing high-frequency *sound waves* through the chest into the heart. The sound waves are then reflected back from the heart, and echoes showing heart structure are displayed on a recording machine. It is a highly useful diagnostic tool in the evaluation of diseases of the valves that separate the heart chambers and diseases of the heart muscle itself.

ECHOENCEPHALOGRAPHY (eh-ko-en-sef-ah-LOG-rah-fe) or ECHOEN-CEPHALOGRAM (eh-ko-en-SEF-ah-lo-gram): An ultrasound recording of the brain (ENCEPHAL/O). Sound waves are beamed at the brain, and the echoes that return to the machine are recorded as graphic tracings. Brain tumors or hematomas (collections of blood) may be detected by abnormal tracings.

ENDOSCOPIC RETROGRADE CHOLANGIOPANCREATOGRAPHY (en-do-SKOP-ik RE-tro-grad kol-an-je-o-pan-kre-ah-TOG-rah-fe): X-ray recording of the bile ducts, pancreas, and pancreatic duct. Dye is injected via a tube through the mouth into the bile and pancreatic ducts. X-rays are then taken.

FLUOROSCOPY (flur-OS-ko-pe): An x-ray procedure that uses a fluorescent screen rather than a photographic plate to show images of the body. X-rays that have passed through the body strike a screen covered with a fluorescent substance that emits yellow-green light. Internal organs can be seen in motion, and the procedure is also used to guide the insertion of catheters.

GALLBLADDER SERIES: See CHOLECYSTOGRAPHY.

HYSTEROSALPINGOGRAPHY (his-ter-o-sal-ping-OG-rah-fe) or HYSTERO-SALPINGOGRAM (his-ter-o-sal-PING-o-gram):   X-ray recording of the uterus and fallopian tubes. Contrast medium is injected through the vagina into the uterus and fallopian tubes, and x-rays are taken to detect blockage or tumor.

INTRAVENOUS PYELOGRAPHY (in-tra-VE-nus pi-eh-LOG-rah-fe):   See PY-ELOGRAPHY.

LOWER GI SERIES: See BARIUM ENEMA.

LYMPHANGIOGRAPHY (limf-an-je-OG-rah-fe) or LYMPHANGIOGRAM (limf-AN-je-o-gram):   X-ray recording of lymph nodes and lymph vessels. After dye is injected into lymphatic vessels in the feet, x-ray pictures are taken of lymph nodes and vessels. The dye travels upward through the lymph vessels of the pelvis, abdomen, and chest and outlines the architecture of nodes in all areas of the body. This procedure is used to detect tumors of the lymph system. It is also called *lymphography*.

LYMPHOGRAPHY (limf-OG-rah-fe):   See LYMPHANGIOGRAPHY.

MAGNETIC RESONANCE IMAGING (mag-NET-ik REZ-o-nans IM-a-jing):   Magnetic waves, not x-rays, are used to create an image of body organs. The images can be taken in several planes of the body — frontal, sagittal (side), and transverse (cross-section) — and are particularly useful for studying brain tumors and tumors of the chest cavity. Also known as *MRI*.

MAMMOGRAPHY (mah-MOG-rah-fe) or MAMMOGRAM (MAM-o-gram):   X-ray recording of the breast. X-rays of low voltage are beamed at the breast and images are produced. The image is recorded on x-ray film or specially coated plates (*xeromammography*). Mammography is used to detect abnormalities in breast tissue.

MYELOGRAPHY (mi-eh-LOG-rah-fe) or MYELOGRAM (MI-eh-lo-gram):   X-ray recording of the spinal cord. X-rays are taken of the fluid-filled space surrounding the spinal cord after dye is injected in the lumbar region of the back. This procedure detects tumors or ruptured, "slipped" disks that lie between the backbones (vertebrae) and press on the spinal cord.

PYELOGRAPHY (pi-eh-LOG-rah-fe) or PYELOGRAM (PI-eh-lo-gram):   X-ray recording of the renal pelvis of the kidney. X-rays are taken of the kidney and other parts of the urinary tract. Dye may be injected intravenously (*intravenous pyelogram*) or through the urethra and urinary bladder (*retrograde pyelogram*). This test is also known as *urography* or a *urogram*.

SMALL BOWEL FOLLOW-THROUGH: See BARIUM SWALLOW.

TOMOGRAPHY (to-MOG-rah-fe) or TOMOGRAM (TO-mo-gram):   X-ray recordings that show an organ in depth. Several pictures ("slices") are taken of an organ by focusing the x-ray machine to blur out certain regions and bring others into sharper focus. Tomograms of the kidney and lung are examples.

ULTRASONOGRAPHY (ul-tra-so-NOG-rah-fe) or ULTRASONOGRAM (ul-tra-SON-o-gram):   Images are produced by beaming *sound waves* into the body and capturing the echoes that bounce off organs. These echoes are then processed to produce an image, not in the sharpest detail, but showing the difference between fluid and solid masses and the general position of organs.

UPPER GI SERIES: See BARIUM SWALLOW.

UROGRAPHY (u-ROG-rah-fe) or UROGRAM (UR-o-gram): See PYELOGRAP

XEROMAMMOGRAPHY (ze-ro-mah-MOG-rah-fe) or XEROMAMMOGRA
ro-MAM-o-gram): See MAMMOGRAPHY.

Nuclear Medicine Scans

In the following diagnostic tests, radioactive material (*radioisotope*) is injected, inhaled, or swallowed and then detected by a scanning device in the organ in which it accumulates. X-rays, ultrasound, or magnetic waves are not used.

BONE SCAN: A radioactive substance is injected intravenously, and its uptake in bones is detected by a scanning device. Tumors in bone can be detected by increased uptake of the radioactive material in the areas of the lesions.

BRAIN SCAN: A radioactive substance is injected intravenously and collects in any lesion that disturbs the natural barrier that exists between blood vessels and normal brain tissue (blood-brain barrier), allowing the radioactive substance to enter the brain tissue. A scanning device detects the presence of the radioactive substance and thus can identify an area of tumor, abscess, or hematoma.

GALLIUM SCAN (GAL-le-um skan): Radioactive gallium (gallium citrate) is injected into the bloodstream and is detected in the body using a scanning device that produces an image of the areas where gallium collects. The gallium collects in areas of certain tumors (Hodgkin's disease, hepatoma, various adenocarcinomas) and in areas of infection.

POSITRON EMISSION TOMOGRAPHY (POS-i-tron e-MISH-un to-MOG-rah-fe): Radioactive substances (oxygen and glucose are used) that release radioactive particles called positrons are injected into the body and travel to specialized areas such as the brain and heart. Because of the way that the positrons are released, cross-sectional color pictures can be made showing the location of the radioactive substance. This test is used to study disorders of the brain and to diagnose strokes, epilepsy, schizophrenia, and migraine headaches. Also known as a *PET scan*.

PULMONARY PERFUSION SCAN (PUL-mon-ar-e per-FU-shun skan): Radioactive particles are injected intravenously and travel rapidly to areas of the lung that are adequately filled with blood. Regions of obstructed blood flow due to tumor, blood clot, swelling, and inflammation can be seen as nonradioactive areas on the scan.

PULMONARY VENTILATION SCAN (PUL-mon-ar-e ven-ti-LA-shun skan): Radioactive gas (xenon-133) is inhaled, and a special camera detects its presence in the lungs. The scan is used to detect lung segments that fail to fill with the radioactive gas. Lack of filling is usually due to diseases that obstruct the bronchial tubes and air sacs. This scan is also used in the evaluation of lung function prior to surgery.

MYOCARDIAL SCAN (mi-o-KAR-de-al skan): A radioactive substance (thallium chloride-201) is injected intravenously and travels to the heart muscle while the patient is at rest or exercising. A special camera shows up areas that have inadequate collection of radioactive substance, such as areas of blocked blood vessels.

THYROID SCAN (THI-royd skan):   A radioactive iodine chemical is injected intravenously and collects in the thyroid gland. A scanning device detects the radioactive substance in the gland, measuring it and producing an image of the gland. The increased or decreased activity of the gland is demonstrated by the gland's capacity to use the radioactive iodine. A thyroid scan is used to evaluate the position, size, and functioning of the thyroid gland.

Clinical Procedures

The following procedures are performed on patients to establish a correct diagnosis of an abnormal condition. In some instances, the procedure may also be used to treat the condition.

ABDOMINOCENTESIS (ab-dom-in-o-sen-TE-sis):   Surgical puncture of the membrane surrounding the abdomen (peritoneum) to remove fluid from the abdominal cavity. Fluid is drained for analysis and to prevent its accumulation in the abdomen. Also known as *paracentesis* or *peritoneocentesis.*

AMNIOCENTESIS (am-ne-o-sen-TE-sis):   Surgical puncture to remove fluid from the sac (amnion) that surrounds the embryo in the uterus. The fluid contains cells from the embryo that can be examined under a microscope.

ASPIRATION (as-peh-RA-shun):   The withdrawal of fluid by suction through a needle or tube.

AUSCULTATION (aw-skul-TA-shun):   Listening for sounds produced within the body. This is most often performed with the aid of a stethoscope to determine the condition of the chest or abdominal organs or to detect pregnancy.

BIOPSY (BI-op-se):   A piece of tissue is removed from the body and examined under a microscope. The tissue is removed by means of a surgical knife, needle aspiration, or an endoscope (using a special forceps-like instrument inserted through a hollow flexible tube). An *excisional biopsy* means that the entire tissue to be examined is removed. An *incisional biopsy* is the removal of only a small amount of tissue, and a *needle biopsy* indicates that the tissue is pierced with a hollow needle and fluid is withdrawn for microscopic examination.

BONE MARROW BIOPSY (bon MAH-ro BI-op-se):   A small amount of bone marrow (soft tissue within bones where blood cells are made) is cored out and examined under a microscope. Often the hip bone (iliac crest) is used, and the biopsy is helpful in determining the number and type of blood cells in the bone marrow.

BRONCHOSCOPY (brong-KOS-ko-pe):   A flexible tube (endoscope) is inserted through the mouth into the windpipe and bronchial tube. The lining of the bronchial tubes can be seen, and tissue can be removed for biopsy.

COLONOSCOPY (ko-lon-OS-ko-pe):   A flexible tube (endoscope) is inserted through the rectum into the large intestine for visual examination of the colon. Biopsy samples can be taken and benign growths, such as polyps, can be removed through the endoscope. The removal of a polyp is called a polypectomy (pol-eh-PEK-to-me).

COLPOSCOPY (kol-POS-ko-pe):   The vaginal walls are held apart with an instrument, and a special microscope (colposcope) is positioned on the outside of the body so that the cervix and vagina can be viewed.

CONIZATION (ko-nih-ZA-shun):   A cone-shaped sample of the uterine cervix moved and examined under the microscope for evidence of cancerous growth. The s shape of the tissue sample allows the pathologist who examines it to cut a thin slice of each of the cervical layers for microscopic examination.

CULDOCENTESIS (kul-do-sen-TE-sis):   A thin, hollow needle is inserted through the vagina into the cul-de-sac, the space between the rectum and the uterus. Fluid is withdrawn and analyzed for evidence of cancerous cells, infection, and blood cells that would indicate bleeding into the cul-de-sac.

CYSTOSCOPY (sis-TOS-ko-pe):   A cystoscope (endoscope) is passed through the urethra into the urinary bladder, and the bladder is visually examined. Tissue may be removed through the cystoscope for biopsy purposes.

DILATION AND CURETTAGE (di-LA-shun and kur-ih-TAJ):   In this procedure, also known as *D and C,* a series of probes of increasing size is inserted through the vagina into the opening of the cervix. The cervix is thus dilated (widened) so that a curette (spoon-shaped instrument) can be inserted to remove tissue from the lining of the uterus. The tissue is then examined under the microscope. Dilation and suction curettage is a procedure used to abort pregnancies up to 12 weeks.

ELECTROCARDIOGRAPHY (e-lek-tro-kar-de-OG-rah-fe):   Electrodes (wires or "leads") are connected to the body by small metal plates, and electric impulses coming from the heart are picked up and recorded by a machine called an electrocardiograph. The *electrocardiogram* (e-lek-tro-KAR-de-o-gram) is the actual record produced, and it is useful in discovering abnormalities in heart rhythms and diagnosing heart disorders. Also called *EKG* or *ECG.*

ELECTROENCEPHALOGRAPHY (e-lek-tro-en-sef-ah-LOG-rah-fe):   Electrodes (wires or "leads") are placed on the scalp to record electricity coming from within the brain. The electroencephalogram is the actual record produced. It is useful in the diagnosis and treatment of epilepsy, tumors, and other brain lesions and in the investigation of other neurological disorders. It is also used to evaluate patients in coma (brain inactivity) and in the study of sleep and its disorders. Also called *EEG.*

ELECTROMYOGRAPHY (e-lek-tro-mi-OG-rah-fe):   This is the process of recording the electrical activity in muscle tissue. Electrical impulses are picked up by needle electrodes that are inserted into muscles. This procedure is useful in detecting injuries and diseases that affect muscles and nerves. Also called *EMG.*

ENDOSCOPY (en-DOS-ko-pe):   A thin, tube-like instrument (endoscope) is used to view the inside of an organ or cavity. It can be inserted through a natural opening such as the mouth or anus or through a surgical incision such as an incision of the abdominal wall. Endoscopes contain bundles of glass fibers that carry light (fiberoptic), and some instruments are equipped with a small forceps-like device that is used to withdraw a sample of tissue for microscopic study (biopsy). Examples of endoscopy are bronchoscopy, colonoscopy, esophagoscopy, gastroscopy, and laparoscopy.

ESOPHAGOSCOPY (eh-sof-ah-GOS-ko-pe):   An endoscope is inserted through the mouth and throat into the esophagus. Visual examination of the esophagus to detect ulcers, tumors, or other lesions is then possible.

EXCISIONAL BIOPSY (ek-SIZ-in-al BI-op-se):   See BIOPSY.

FROZEN SECTION (FRO-zen SEK-shun): This technique is used to prepare a biopsy sample for examination. The tissue is taken from the operating room to the pathology laboratory and frozen. It is then thinly sliced and examined under the microscope to determine if the sample is benign or malignant (cancerous).

GASTROSCOPY (gas-TROS-ko-pe): Visual examination of the stomach and upper part of the small intestine using an endoscope (gastroscope) that is inserted through the mouth, throat (pharynx), and esophagus.

HOLTER ECG RECORDING (HOL-ter ECG re-KOR-ding): A method in which prolonged (usually 24 hour) electrocardiographic records are made on a portable tape recorder while the patient engages in normal daily activities. It is useful in detecting and managing abnormalities in heart rhythms. Also called *Holter monitoring.*

HYSTEROSCOPY (his-ter-OS-ko-pe): Visual examination of the uterus using an endoscope that is inserted through the vagina and cervix.

INCISIONAL BIOPSY (in-SIZ-in-al BI-op-se): See BIOPSY.

LAPAROSCOPY (lah-pah-ROS-ko-pe): Visual examination of the abdomen using an endoscope. After the patient receives a local anesthetic, the laparoscope is inserted through an incision in the abdominal wall. This procedure gives the doctor a view of the abdominal cavity, the surface of the liver and spleen, and the pelvic region. The laparoscope can be used to cut and burn (cauterize) the ends of the fallopian tubes to produce sterilization (inability to reproduce) in a female. Also called *peritoneoscopy.*

LARYNGOSCOPY (lah-rin-GOS-ko-pe): Visual examination of the voice box (larynx). A laryngoscope (endoscope) transmits a magnified image of the larynx through a system of lenses and mirrors. The procedure is used to reveal tumors and to explain changes in the voice. Samples of sputum and biopsies may also be obtained by using brushes or forceps attached to the laryngoscope.

MEDIASTINOSCOPY (me-de-ah-sti-NOS-ko-pe): Visual examination of the mediastinum (space in the chest between the lungs and in front of the heart). A mediastinoscope is inserted through a small surgical incision in the neck while the patient is under anesthesia. This procedure is used to biopsy lymph nodes and examine other structures within the mediastinum.

NEEDLE BIOPSY (NE-dl BI-op-se): See BIOPSY.

PALPATION (pal-PA-shun): Examination by touch. This is a technique of physical examination by which a doctor uses his or her hands to feel underlying tissues and organs through the skin.

PAP SMEAR (pap smer): This test for cervical cancer was developed by the late Dr. George Papanicolaou. A physician inserts a cotton swab or wooden spatula into the vagina to obtain a sample of cells from the outer surface of the cervix (the neck of the uterus). The cells are then smeared on a glass slide, preserved, and sent to the laboratory for microscopic examination.

PARACENTESIS (pah-rah-sen-TE-sis): See ABDOMINOCENTESIS.

PERCUSSION (per-KUSH-un): Striking a part of the body with short, sharp blows of the fingers to determine the size, density, and position of the underlying parts by the sound obtained. Percussion is most commonly used on the chest to examine the heart and lungs.

PERITONEOCENTESIS (peh-rih-to-ne-o-sen-TE-sis): See ABDOMINOCENTESIS.

PERITONEOSCOPY (peh-rih-to-ne-OS-ko-pe): See LAPAROSCOPY.

PROCTOSIGMOIDOSCOPY (prok-to-sig-moy-DOS-ko-pe): Visual examina
the rectum and the sigmoid colon. A proctoscope or sigmoidoscope is inserted through the
anus to examine the first 10 to 12 inches of the rectum and colon. Also known as *sigmoidoscopy*,
this procedure can demonstrate growths in the region examined.

**PULMONARY FUNCTION STUDY (PUL-mo-nah-re FUNG-shun STUH-
de):** Measurement of the air taken into and exhaled from the lungs by means of an instrument called a *spirometer*.

SIGMOIDOSCOPY (sig-moy-DOS-ko-pe): See PROCTOSIGMOIDOSCOPY.

THORACENTESIS (thor-ah-sen-TE-sis): Surgical puncture of the chest to remove
fluid from the space surrounding the lungs (pleural cavity). After injection of a local anesthetic, a hollow needle is inserted through the skin and muscles of the back and into the space
between the lungs and the chest wall. Fluid is then withdrawn by applying suction. Excess
fluid (called a pleural effusion) may be a sign of infection or malignancy. This procedure, also
called *thoracocentesis*, may be used for diagnostic studies, to drain pleural effusions, or to
re-expand a collapsed lung (atelectasis).

THORACOCENTESIS (thor-ah-ko-sen-TE-sis): See THORACENTESIS.

THORACOSCOPY (tho-rah-KOS-ko-pe): Visual examination of the chest using an
endoscope. The endoscope is inserted through an incision in the chest and the surface of the
lungs can be examined.

Laboratory Tests

The following laboratory tests are performed on samples of a patient's blood, *plasma*
(fluid portion of the blood), *serum* (plasma minus clotting proteins and produced after blood
has clotted), urine, feces, *sputum* (mucus coughed up from the lungs), *cerebrospinal fluid* (fluid
within the spaces around the spinal cord and brain), and skin.

ACID PHOSPHATASE (AH-sid FOS-fah-tas): This test measures the amount of an
enzyme called acid phosphatase in serum. Enzyme levels are elevated in cancer of the prostate
gland that has metastasized. Moderate elevations of this enzyme occur in some bone diseases
and in invasion of bone by breast cancer cells.

ALBUMIN (al-BU-min): Albumin (protein) can be measured in serum and in urine. A
decrease of albumin in serum may indicate disease of the kidneys, malnutrition, or liver
disease or may be due to extensive burns. High levels of albumin in the urine may indicate poor
functioning of the kidneys.

ALKALINE PHOSPHATASE (AL-kah-lin FOS-fah-tas): This test measures the
amount of an enzyme called alkaline phosphatase in serum. Levels are elevated in certain liver
abnormalities, such as hepatitis and cancer, and in bone diseases, such as Paget's disease and
cancer involving the bone. Also called *alk phos*.

ALPHA-FETOPROTEIN (al-fa-fe-to-PRO-ten): This is a test for the presence of a
protein called alpha-globulin in serum. It is normally present in the serum of the fetus, infant,
and pregnant woman. High levels are found in patients with cancer of the liver and other
malignancies (most testicular and some ovarian cancers). In fetuses with abnormalities of

development of the spinal cord and brain, the protein leaks into the fluid surrounding the fetus (amniotic fluid) and is an indicator of spina bifida (incomplete development of the spinal cord) and anencephaly (lack of brain development).

BENCE JONES PROTEIN (BENS jonz PRO-ten):   This test measures the presence of the Bence Jones protein in the serum or urine. The Bence Jones protein is a fragment of the protein produced by cancerous bone marrow cells (myeloma cells). Normally it is not found in either blood or urine, but in multiple myeloma (malignant condition of the bone marrow) high levels of Bence Jones protein are detected in urine and serum.

BILIRUBIN (bil-eh-RU-bin):   This test measures the amount of bilirubin, an orange-brown pigment, in the serum or urine. Its presence in high concentrations in serum and urine causes jaundice (yellow coloration of the skin) and may indicate disease of the liver, obstruction of bile ducts, or a type of anemia that leads to excessive destruction of red blood cells.

BLOOD CULTURE (blud KUL-chur):   In this test, a sample of blood is added to a special medium (food) that promotes the growth of microorganisms. The medium is then examined under the microscope for evidence of bacteria or other microbes.

BLOOD UREA NITROGEN (blud u-RE-ah NI-tro-jen):   This test measures the amount of urea (a nitrogen-containing waste material) in the serum or plasma. A high level of urea indicates poor kidney function, since it is the kidney's job to remove urea from the bloodstream and filter it into urine.

CALCIUM (KAL-se-um):   This test measures the amount of calcium (an important mineral found in bones and blood) in the serum, plasma, or whole blood. Low blood levels are associated with abnormal functioning of nerves and muscles, and high blood levels may indicate loss of calcium from bones, excessive intake of calcium, disease of the parathyroid glands, or cancer.

CARCINOEMBRYONIC ANTIGEN (kar-sih-no-em-bre-ON-ik AN-ti-jen):   This is a plasma test for a protein normally found in the blood of human fetuses and produced in healthy adults only in a very small amount, if at all. High levels of this antigen in the blood may be a sign of one of a variety of cancers, especially cancer of the colon or pancreas. Also called *CEA*.

CEREBROSPINAL FLUID (seh-re-bro-SPI-nal FLU-id):   Chemical tests are performed on specimens of cerebrospinal fluid (*CSF*) removed from between membranes surrounding the spinal cord. The fluid is tested for protein content, sugar, and blood cells. CSF is also cultured to detect microorganisms. Abnormal conditions such as meningitis (inflammation of membranes around the spinal cord and brain), brain tumor, and encephalitis (inflammation of the brain) can be detected by CSF analysis.

CHOLESTEROL (ko-LES-ter-ol):   This test measures the amount of cholesterol (a substance found in animal fats and oils, egg yolks, and milk) in the serum or plasma. Normal values vary for age and diet; levels above 200 mg/dl indicate a need for further testing and efforts to reduce cholesterol level, since high levels are associated with hardening of arteries and heart disease. Blood can also be tested for the presence of a lipoprotein substance that is a combination of cholesterol and protein. High levels of HDL (high density lipoprotein) cholesterol in the blood are thought to be beneficial, since HDL cholesterol promotes the removal and excretion of excess cholesterol from the body, while high levels of low density lipoprotein (LDL) are dangerous.

CREATINE KINASE (KRE-ah-tin KI-nas):   This test measures the amount of an enzyme called creatine kinase (*CK*) in serum. It is normally found in heart muscle, brain tissue, and skeletal muscle. The presence of one form of creatine kinase in the blood is strongly indicative of recent myocardial infarction (heart attack), since the enzyme is released from the heart muscle when the muscle is damaged or dying.

CREATININE (kre-AT-ih-nin): This test measures the amount of creatinine, a nitrogen-containing waste material, in serum or plasma. If levels are high, the kidney is not able to effectively remove the creatinine from the blood and filter it into urine.

CREATININE CLEARANCE (kre-AT-ih-nin KLER-ans): This test measures the rate at which creatinine is cleared (filtered) from the blood. If creatinine clearance is low, it indicates that the kidneys are not functioning effectively to clear creatinine from the bloodstream and filter it into urine.

CULTURE (KUL-chur): This test measures the growth of microorganisms or of living cells in a special laboratory medium (fluid, solid, or semisolid material). In *culture and sensitivity* tests, culture plates containing a specific microorganism are prepared, and antibiotic-containing disks are applied to the culture surface. Following overnight incubation, the area surrounding the disk (where growth of microorganisms is held back) is measured to determine if the antibiotic is effective against the specific organism.

ELECTROLYTES (e-LEK-tro-litz): Electrolytes are substances that, when dissolved in water, break apart into electrically charged particles, capable of conducting an electric current. Examples of electrolytes are sodium (Na^+), potassium (K^+), calcium (Ca^{++}), magnesium (Mg^{++}), and chloride (Cl^-). Tests are done on serum (cell-free portion of the blood) to determine the concentration of electrolytes, which should be present at all times for the proper functioning of cells. An electrolyte imbalance occurs when the serum concentration of an electrolyte is either too high or too low. Calcium imbalance can affect the bones, kidneys, and gastrointestinal tract and neuromuscular activity. Sodium affects blood pressure, nerve functioning, and fluid levels surrounding cells. Potassium affects the heart and muscles.

ELECTROPHORESIS (e-lek-tro-fo-RE-sis): See PROTEIN ELECTROPHORESIS.

ELISA (eh-LI-zah): This is a laboratory assay (test) for the presence in a patient's blood of antibodies to the AIDS virus. If a patient tests positive, it is likely that his or her blood contains the AIDS virus (called HIV or human immunodeficiency virus). The presence of the virus causes white blood cells to make antibodies that are detected by the ELISA assay. This is the first test done to detect AIDS infection and is followed by a western blot test to confirm the results. ELISA is an acronym for *enzyme-linked immunosorbent assay*.

ERYTHROCYTE SEDIMENTATION RATE (eh-RITH-ro-sit sed-ih-men-TA-shun rat): This test measures the rate at which red blood cells in well-mixed venous blood settle to the bottom (sediment) of a test tube. If the rate of sedimentation is markedly rapid, it may indicate inflammatory conditions, such as rheumatoid arthritis, or conditions that produce excessive quantities of proteins in the blood. Also called *ESR* or *Sed. rate*.

ESTRADIOL (es-tra-DI-ol): This is a test for the concentration of estradiol, which is a form of estrogen (female hormone), in serum, plasma, or urine.

ESTROGEN RECEPTOR ASSAY (ES-tro-jen re-SEP-tor AS-a): This test, performed at the time of a biopsy, determines if a sample of tumor contains an estrogen receptor protein. The protein, if present on breast cancer cells, combines with estrogen, allowing estrogen to promote the growth of the tumor. Thus, if an estrogen receptor assay test is positive (the protein is present) then treatment with an anti-estrogen drug would slow down tumor growth. If the assay is negative (the protein is not present), then the tumor would not be affected by anti-estrogen drug treatment.

GLOBULIN (GLOB-u-lin):   Globulins are proteins, made by cells of the immune system, that bind to and destroy foreign substances. These proteins are found in plasma (fluid portion of the blood) and can be analyzed and measured in serum (plasma minus the proteins that aid in clotting). The procedure that is used to separate the various globulins is called *protein electrophoresis.*

GLUCOSE (GLU-kos):   This test measures the amount of glucose (a sugar and the main source of energy of body cells) in the serum and plasma. High levels of glucose (hyperglycemia) may indicate abnormal conditions, such as diabetes mellitus. Glucose is also measured in urine (glycosuria), and its presence also indicates diabetes.

GLUCOSE TOLERANCE TEST (GLU-kos TOL-er-ans test):   In the first part of this test, a blood sample is taken after the patient has fasted. Then, a solution of glucose is given by mouth. One-half hour after the glucose is taken, blood and urine samples are obtained, and they are collected every hour for 4 to 5 hours. The test determines the way the body uses glucose and may indicate abnormal conditions such as diabetes mellitus, hypoglycemia (low blood sugar), and liver or adrenal gland dysfunction.

HEMATOCRIT (he-MAT-o-krit):   This test measures the percentage of red blood cells (erythrocytes) in the blood. The normal value is 40 to 50 per cent in males and 37 to 47 per cent in females. A low hematocrit often indicates anemia (deficiency of red blood cells or hemoglobin). Also called *Hct.*

HEMOGLOBIN ASSAY (HE-mo-glo-bin AS-a):   This test measures the concentration of hemoglobin (a blood protein in red blood cells) in blood. The normal blood hemoglobin values are 13.5 to 18.0 gm/dl in adult males and 12.0 to 16.0 in adult females. Also called *Hgb.*

HUMAN CHORIONIC GONADOTROPIN (HU-man kor-e-ON-ik go-nad-o-TRO-pin):   This test measures the concentration of the hormone human chorionic gonadotropin (hCG) in urine. It can be detected in urine within days after fertilization (union) of egg and sperm cells. The measurement of hCG in urine is commonly referred to as the pregnancy test.

IMMUNOASSAY (im-u-no-AS-a):   This method tests blood and urine for the concentration of various chemicals, such as hormones, drugs, or proteins. The technique makes use of the immunological reaction between antigens and antibodies, so it is referred to as an immunoassay. An assay is a determination of the amount of any particular substance in a mixture.

LE PREP: This is a test of a patient's white blood cells for their reaction to normal blood cells. Patients with lupus erythematosus have abnormal white blood cells (called L.E. cells) that have engulfed and absorbed other cells.

OCCULT BLOOD TEST (o-KULT blud test):   A small sample of stool is tested for otherwise inapparent ("occult" means "hidden") traces of blood. The sample is smeared on a slide and examined under the microscope.

PKU TEST: This test determines if the urine of a newborn baby contains substances called phenylketones. If so, the condition is called phenylketonuria (PKU). Phenylketonuria occurs when infants are born missing a specific enzyme. This enzyme normally helps convert one amino acid to another in the bloodstream. If the enzyme is missing and the PKU test positive, excessive amounts of an amino acid (phenylalanine) accumulate in the blood, affecting the brain and causing mental retardation. To prevent this from happening, the infant with PKU is placed on a special diet that prevents accumulation of the specific amino acid in the bloodstream.

PLATELET COUNT (PLAT-let kownt):   This test determines the number of clotting cells (platelets or thrombocytes) in a sample of blood.

POTASSIUM (po-TAHS-e-um):   This test measures the concentration of potassium (a mineral electrolyte) in serum. Potassium (K^+) combines with other minerals (such as calcium) in the body and is an important chemical for the proper functioning of muscles, especially heart muscle.

PROGESTERONE RECEPTOR ASSAY (pro-JES-ter-on re-SEP-tor AS-a):   This test determines if a sample of tumor contains a progesterone receptor protein. If positive, it identifies tumor that would be responsive to anti-progesterone hormone therapy.

PROTEIN ELECTROPHORESIS (PRO-ten e-lek-tro-for-E-sis):   This procedure separates proteins using an electric current. The material tested, such as serum, containing various proteins, is placed on paper or gel or in liquid and, under the influence of an electric current, the proteins separate (-PHORESIS means separation) so that they can be identified and measured. Also known as *serum protein electrophoresis*.

PROTHROMBIN TIME (pro-THROM-bin tim):   This test measures the activity of factors in the blood that participate in clotting. Deficiency of any of these factors can lead to a prolonged prothrombin time and difficulty in blood clotting. The test is important as a monitor for patients who are taking anticoagulants, substances that block the activity of blood clotting factors, and as a side effect, increase the risk of bleeding.

RED BLOOD CELL (RBC) COUNT: This test counts the number of red blood cells (erythrocytes) in a sample of blood. A low red blood cell count indicates anemia.

RHEUMATOID FACTOR (RU-mah-toyd FAK-ter):   This test detects an abnormal protein (rheumatoid factor) present in the serum of patients with rheumatoid arthritis.

SERUM GLUTAMIC-OXALOACETIC TRANSAMINASE (SE-rum glu-TAM-ik oks-al-ah-SE-tik trans-AM-in-as):   This test, also called *SGOT* or *AST*, measures the amount of an enzyme (serum glutamate oxaloacetate transaminase) in serum. The enzyme is normally present, but when there is damage to heart or liver cells, it is produced by the damaged tissue and accumulates in the blood.

SERUM GLUTAMATE PYRUVIC-TRANSAMINASE (SE-rum GLU-ta-mat pi-RU-vik trans-AM-in-as):   This test, also called *SGPT* or *ALT*, measures the amount of an enzyme (serum glutamate pyruvate transaminase) in serum. The enzyme is normally in the blood but accumulates in abnormally high amounts when there is acute damage to liver cells.

SERUM PROTEIN ELECTROPHORESIS (SE-rum PRO-ten e-lek-tro-for-E-sis):   See PROTEIN ELECTROPHORESIS.

SKIN TESTS: In these tests, substances are applied to the skin or injected under the skin, and the reaction of immune cells in the skin is observed. These tests detect a person's sensitivity to substances such as dust or pollen. They can also indicate if a person has been exposed to the bacteria that cause tuberculosis or diphtheria.

SPUTUM TEST (SPU-tum test):   This test examines mucus that is coughed up from the patient's lungs. The sputum is examined microscopically and chemically and cultured for the presence of microorganisms.

THYROID CHEMISTRIES (THI-royd KEM-is-trez):   These tests measure the levels of thyroid hormones, such as thyroxine (T_4) and triiodothyronine (T_3) in serum. Thyroid-stimulating hormone (TSH), which is produced by the pituitary gland and stimulates the release of T_4 and T_3 from the thyroid gland, can also be measured in the serum.

TRIGLYCERIDES (tri-GLIS-er-idz):   This test determines the amount of triglycerides (fats) in the serum. Elevated triglycerides are considered an important risk factor for the development of heart disease.

URIC ACID (UR-ik AS-id):   This test measures the amount of uric acid (a nitrogen-containing waste material) in the serum and urine. High levels of uric acid are found in a patient with a type of arthritis called gout. In gout, uric acid accumulates as crystals in joints and tissues.

URINALYSIS (u-rih-NAL-ih-sis):   Analysis of urine as an aid in the diagnosis of disease. Routine urinalysis (*U/A*) consists of observing any unusual color or odor, determining specific gravity (amount of materials dissolved in urine), chemical tests (for protein, sugar, acetone), and microscopic examination for bacteria, blood cells, and casts (molds of substances that collect in kidney tubules).

WESTERN BLOT (WES-tern blot):   This test is more specific than the ELISA to detect infection by the AIDS virus. A patient's serum is mixed with purified proteins from the AIDS virus and the reaction is examined. If the patient has made antibodies to the AIDS virus, those antibodies will react with the purified AIDS virus proteins, and the test will be positive.

WHITE BLOOD CELL (WBC) COUNT: This test determines the number of white blood cells (leukocytes) in the blood. Higher than normal counts may indicate the presence of infection or leukemia.

APPENDIX III

ABBREVIATIONS AND SYMBOLS

Abbreviations

ABO	Three main blood types
a.c.	Before meals *(ante cibum)*
ACTH	Adrenocorticotropic hormone (secreted by the pituitary gland)
ADH	Antidiuretic hormone (secreted by the pituitary gland)
ad lib	Freely as desired (ad libitum)
AIDS	Acquired immune deficiency syndrome
ALL	Acute lymphocytic (lymphoblastic) leukemia
alk phos	Alkaline phosphatase (enzyme elevated in liver disease)
ALS	Amyotrophic lateral sclerosis (Lou Gehrig's disease)
ALT	Alanine transaminase (enzyme elevated in liver disease); see SGPT
AML	Acute myelocytic leukemia
AP	Anteroposterior (front to back)
A & P	Auscultation and percussion
aq	Water *(aqua)*
ASHD	Arteriosclerotic heart disease
AST	Aspartate aminotransferase (elevated in liver and heart disease); see SGOT
Ba	Barium
BaE	Barium enema
B-cells	White blood cells (lymphocytes) produced in the bone marrow
b/f, b/m	Black female, black male
b.i.d.	Twice a day *(bis in die)*
BM	Bowel movement; bone marrow
BP	Blood pressure
BPH	Benign prostatic hyperplasia (hypertrophy)
Broncho	Bronchoscopy
BUN	Blood urea nitrogen (test of kidney function)
Bx	Biopsy
$\bar{c}$	With *(cum)*
C1, C2	First, second cervical vertebra
Ca	Calcium; cancer or carcinoma
CABG	Coronary artery bypass graft
CAD	Coronary artery disease
CAPD	Continuous ambulatory peritoneal dialysis (method of cleansing the body of wastes when the kidney is not functioning)
caps	Capsules
CBC	Complete blood count
cc	Cubic centimeter (1/1000 liter)

CCU	Coronary care unit
Chemo	Chemotherapy
CHF	Congestive heart failure
cm	Centimeter (1/100 meter)
CML	Chronic myelogenous leukemia
CNS	Central nervous system
CO_2	Carbon dioxide (a gas produced by cells and excreted by the lungs)
COPD	Chronic obstructive pulmonary disease (chronic bronchitis, emphysema)
CPR	Cardiopulmonary resuscitation
crit	See HCT
C-section	Cesarean section
CSF	Cerebrospinal fluid
CT	Computed tomography (see CT SCAN)
CT scan	Computed axial tomography (x-ray in a cross-sectional view)
CVA	Cerebrovascular accident (stroke)
CXR	Chest x-ray
D/c	Discontinue; discharge
D & C	Dilation and curettage (widening and scraping the lining of the uterus)
Derm	Dermatology
DES	Diethylstilbestrol (form of estrogen; known to cause defects in children whose mothers have taken it during pregnancy)
diff	Differential (count of numbers of different white blood cells)
dil	Dilute
DNA	Deoxyribonucleic acid (genetic material in a cell)
DOB	Date of birth
DT	Delirium tremens (mental disturbance caused by alcohol withdrawal)
Dx	Diagnosis
EBV	Epstein-Barr virus (cause of mononucleosis)
ECG	Electrocardiogram
ECT	Electroconvulsive therapy (used in treatment of mental disorders)
EEG	Electroencephalogram
EGD	Esophagogastroduodenoscopy (visual examination of the esophagus, stomach, and duodenum)
EKG	Electrocardiogram
EMG	Electromyogram
ENT	Ear, nose, and throat
Eos	Eosinophils (a type of white blood cell)
ER	Emergency room; estrogen receptor
ERT	Estrogen replacement therapy

ESR	Erythrocyte sedimentation rate; See SED. RATE
ESWL	Extracorporeal shock wave lithotripsy
exc	Excision
FBS	Fasting blood sugar
FDA	Food and Drug Administration
Fe	Iron
FH	Family history
FHT	Fetal heart tones
FSH	Follicle-stimulating hormone (secreted by the pituitary gland)
F/u	Follow-up
5-FU	5-Fluorouracil (a drug used in cancer chemotherapy)
FUO	Fever of unknown origin
Ga	Gallium (radioactive substance used in studies to locate tumors)
GB	Gallbladder
GBS	Gallbladder series (x-rays)
GH	Growth hormone (secreted by the pituitary gland)
GI	Gastrointestinal
Gm, gm	Gram
Grav. 1,2,3	First, second, third pregnancy
gt, gtt	Drops
GTT	Glucose tolerance test
GU	Genitourinary
Gyn	Gynecology
H	Hydrogen
h	Hour
Hb (Hgb)	Hemoglobin
HCG	Human chorionic gonadotropin (hormone secreted by the placenta during pregnancy)
HCl	Hydrochloric acid
Hct	Hematocrit (percentage of red blood cells in a given volume of blood)
HD	Hemodialysis (use of an artificial kidney machine)
HDL	High density lipoproteins (associated with decreased incidence of coronary artery disease)
Hg	Mercury
Hgb	Hemoglobin (protein within red blood cells)
hGH	Human growth hormone (see GH)
HIV	Human immunodeficiency virus
h/o	History of
H_2O	Water
h.s.	At bedtime *(hora somni)*

HSG	Hysterosalpingogram (x-ray of the uterus and fallopian tubes)
hx	History
I	Iodine
ICU	Intensive care unit
IDDM	Insulin-dependent diabetes mellitus (juvenile diabetes, type I)
IM	Intramuscular
INH	Isoniazid hydrochloride (drug used to treat tuberculosis)
inj	Injection
I & O	Intake and output (measurement of patient's fluids)
I.Q.	Intelligence quotient
IUD	Intrauterine device (contraceptive device)
IV	Intravenous
IVC	Intravenous cholangiogram (x-ray of bile ducts)
IVP	Intravenous pyelogram (x-ray of the kidney and urinary tract)
K^+	Potassium (an electrolyte)
Kg	Kilogram (1000 grams)
KUB	Kidney, ureter, bladder (x-ray of the abdomen without using dye)
L	Liter (1.05 quarts); lower
Ⓛ	Left
L1, L2	First, second lumbar vertebra
LA	Left atrium (chamber of the heart)
Lat	Lateral (side)
LB	Large bowel
LD, LDH	Lactic dehydrogenase (associated with damage to heart muscle)
LDL	Low density lipoproteins (high levels associated with heart disease)
LE	Lupus erythematosus (a disorder of skin, connective tissue, and joints)
LLQ	Left lower quadrant of the abdomen
LMP	Last menstrual period
LP	Lumbar puncture
LUQ	Left upper quadrant of the abdomen
LV	Left ventricle (lower heart chamber)
lymphs	Lymphocytes (white blood cells)
lytes	Electrolytes
m	Meter
MCH	Mean corpuscular hemoglobin (amount of hemoglobin in each red blood cell)
MCHC	Mean corpuscular hemoglobin concentration (amount of hemoglobin per unit of blood)
MCV	Mean corpuscular volume (measurement of the size of an individual red blood cell)

mets	Metastases
mg	Milligram (1/1000 gram)
Mg^{++}	Magnesium (an electrolyte)
MH	Marital history
MI	Myocardial infarction (heart attack)
ml	Milliliter (1/1000 liter)
mm	Millimeter (1/1000 meter: 0.039 inch)
mm Hg	Millimeters of mercury (measurement of blood pressure)
mon, mono	Monocytes (white blood cells)
MRI	Magnetic resonance imaging
MS	Multiple sclerosis
MTX	Methotrexate (drug used in cancer chemotherapy)
MVP	Mitral valve prolapse (abnormality of a heart valve)
Myop	Myopia (nearsightedness)
Na^+	Sodium (an electrolyte)
NB	Newborn
NED	No evidence of disease
neg	Negative
neuro	Neurology
NG tube	Nasogastric tube
NIDDM	Non–insulin-dependent diabetes mellitus (adult-onset diabetes; type II)
NKA	No known allergies
NPO	Nothing by mouth *(nulla per os)*
NTP	Normal temperature and pressure
O_2	Oxygen
OB	Obstetrics
Occ. Th.	Occupational Therapy
OCG	Oral cholecystogram
OD	Right eye *(oculus dexter)*
op	Operation
OPD	Outpatient department
Ophth	Ophthalmology
OR	Operating room
Ortho	Orthopedics; orthopaedics
OS	Left eye *(oculus sinister)*
os	Mouth
OU	Each eye *(oculus uterque)*
OV	Office visit
P	Pulse; phosphorus

PA	Posteroanterior (from back to front)
PAC	Premature atrial contraction (abnormal heart rhythm)
$PaCO_2$	Pressure of carbon dioxide in the blood; also written PCO_2
palp	Palpable; palpation (to examine by touch)
PaO_2	Pressure of oxygen in the blood
Pap smear	Papanicolaou smear (microscopic examination of cells from the cervix and vagina)
Para 1, 2, 3	Unipara, bipara, tripara (indicating a woman having one, two, and three children)
PAT	Paroxysmal atrial tachycardia (abnormal heart rhythm)
Path	Pathology
p.c.	After meals (*post cibum*)
PD	Peritoneal dialysis
PDN	Private duty nurse
PE	Physical examination
Ped	Pediatrics
PEG	Percutaneous endoscopic gastrostomy (new opening into the stomach from the outside of the body); pneumoencephalogram
PERLA	See PERRLA
PERRLA	Pupils equal, round, and reactive to light and accommodation
PE tube	Ventilating tube for eardrum
pH	Hydrogen ion concentration (measurement of the acidity or alkalinity of a solution)
PH	Past history
PI	Present illness
PID	Pelvic inflammatory disease (inflammation of the fallopian tubes)
PKU	Phenylketonuria (infants lack an enzyme, leading to accumulation of phenylketones in the urine; hereditary condition)
PM	Post mortem; afternoon (*post meridian*)
PMN	Polymorphonuclear leukocytes (white blood cells)
p/o	postoperative
p.o.	orally (*per os*)
polys	Polymorphonuclear leukocytes (white blood cells)
poplit	popliteal (behind the knee)
pos	Positive
post-op	After operation
PP	After meals (*post prandial*)
PPD	Purified protein derivative (skin test for tuberculosis)
pre-op	Before operation
prep	Prepare for

p.r.n. (PRN)	As often as necessary *(pro re nata)*
procto	Proctoscopy (visual examination of the anus and rectum)
Pro. time	Prothrombin time (test of blood clotting)
Psych	Psychiatry
PT	Physical therapy
pt	Patient
PTA	Prior to admission
PTCA	Percutaneous transluminal coronary angioplasty (balloon angioplasty)
PTR	Patient to return
PVC	Premature ventricular contraction (abnormal heart rhythm)
q	Each *(quaque)*
q.d.	Each day *(quaque die)*
q.h.	Each hour *(quaque hora)*
q2h	Each two hours *(quaque secunda hora)*
q.i.d.	Four times a day *(quater in die)*
q.n.	Each night *(quaque nox)*
q.n.s.	Quantity not sufficient *(quaque non status)*
qsuff	As much as needed
R, r, rt	Right
Ⓡ	Right
RA	Rheumatoid arthritis; right atrium (chamber of the heart)
Ra	Radium
RAtx	Radiation therapy
RBC, rbc	Red blood cell
REC	Alive, with evidence of recurrence (after remission)
REM	Alive, no evidence of residual cancer (remission)
req	Requested
resp	Respirations
RHD	Rheumatic heart disease
RIA	Radioimmunoassay (laboratory procedure to measure minute quantities of substances)
RLQ	Right lower quadrant of the abdomen
R/O	Rule out
ROM	Range of motion
ROS	Review of systems
RT	Radiation therapy
RUQ	Right upper quadrant of the abdomen
RR	Recovery room
RV	Right ventricle (chamber of the heart)
Rx	Treatment

s̄	Without *(sine)*
S1, S2	First, second sacral vertebra
S-A node	Sino-atrial node (region of electrical conduction within the heart muscle; pacemaker of the heart)
SBFT	Small bowel follow-through (x-ray study of the small intestine)
Sed. rate	Sedimentation rate (time it takes red blood cells to settle out of blood); also known as *ESR*
segs	Segmented cells (white blood cells)
s̄. gl.	without glasses (correction)
SGOT (AST)	Serum glutamic-oxaloacetic transminase (high blood levels of this enzyme are associated with liver and heart disease)
SGPT (ALT)	Serum glutamic-pyruvic transaminase (high blood levels of this enzyme are associated with liver disease)
SH	Serum hepatitis; social history
sig	Let it be labeled
SLE	Systemic lupus erythematosus (disease of skin and connective tissue)
SOAP	Charting *subjective* data (symptoms perceived by patient), *objective* data (exam findings), *assessment* (evaluation of condition), *plan* (goals for treatment)
SOB	Shortness of breath
sol	Solution
S/P	Status post (previous disease condition)
Staph	*Staphylococcus* (bacterium)
stat	Immediately *(statim)*
Strep	*Streptococcus* (bacterium)
STS	Test for syphilis
Subcu	Subcutaneous (under the skin)
Sub q	See SUBCU
supp	Suppository
Sx	Symptoms
T	Temperature
T1, T2	First, second thoracic vertebra
T_3	Triiodothyronine (a hormone from the thyroid gland)
T_4	Thyroxine (a hormone from the thyroid gland)
T & A	Tonsillectomy and adenoidectomy
tab	Tablet
TAH	Total abdominal hysterectomy
TB	Tuberculosis
T-cells	Lymphocytes (white blood cells) originating in the thymus gland
T & C	Type and cross-match

TIA	Transient ischemic attack (interruption of proper blood supply to the brain)
t.i.d.	Three times daily *(ter in die)*
TLC	Total lung capacity
TNM	Tumor, nodes, and metastases; used in staging cancer spread
tomos	Tomograms (series of x-rays to show an organ in depth)
TPN	Total parenteral nutrition (intravenous feeding)
TPR	Temperature, pulse, and respiration
Trig	Triglycerides
TSH	Thyroid-stimulating hormone (produced by the pituitary gland)
TUR, TURP	Transurethral resection of the prostate gland
TVH	Total vaginal hysterectomy
Tx	treatment
U	Unit
U/A, Ua	Urinalysis
UGI	Upper gastrointestinal (x-rays of the digestive tract)
umb	Navel *(umbilicus)*
ung	Ointment
U/O	Urine output
URI	Upper respiratory infection
Urol	Urology
u/s	Ultrasound
UTI	Urinary tract infection
UV	Ultraviolet
VA	Visual acuity (ability to see)
vag	Vagina, vaginal
VCU	Voiding cystourethrogram (x-ray of the urinary tract taken while urinating)
VD	Venereal disease
VDRL	Venereal disease research laboratory (a test for syphilis)
VF	Visual field
Vit	Vitamin
VLDL	Very low density lipoproteins
VSD	Ventricular septal defect (structural abnormality within the heart)
V tach, V.T.	Ventricular tachycardia (abnormal heart rhythm)
WBC	White blood count
wbc	White blood cell
W/C	Wheel chair
wd	Wound
w/f, w/m	White female, white male

WNL	Within normal limits
WT, wt.	Weight
w/u	Workup
y/o	Year(s) old

Symbols

=	Equal
≠	Unequal
+	Positive
−	Negative
↑	Above, increase
↓	Below, decrease
♀	Female
♂	Male
→	To (in direction of)
>	Is greater than
<	Is less than
1°, 2°	Primary, secondary to
ʒ	Dram
℥	Ounce

GLOSSARY OF MEDICAL TERMS

Pronunciation of each term is given with its meaning.* The syllable that gets the accent is in CAPITAL LETTERS. Terms in SMALL CAPITAL LETTERS are defined elsewhere in the glossary.

ABDOMEN (AB-do-men):   space below the chest, containing organs such as the stomach, liver, intestines, and gallbladder. Also called the abdominal cavity, the abdomen lies between the diaphragm and the pelvis (hip bone).

ABDOMINAL (ab-DOM-i-nal):   pertaining to the abdomen.

ABDOMINAL CAVITY (ab-DOM-i-nal KAV-i-te):   see ABDOMEN.

ABNORMAL (ab-NOR-mal):   pertaining to being away (AB-) from the norm; irregular.

ACUTE (a-KUT):   sharp, sudden, intense for a short period of time.

ADENITIS (ad-eh-NI-tis):   inflammation of a gland.

ADENOCARCINOMA (ah-deh-no-kar-sih-NO-mah):   cancerous tumor of glandular cells.

ADENOIDS (AD-eh-noidz):   enlarged lymphatic tissue in the upper part of the throat near the nasal passageways.

ADENOIDECTOMY (ah-deh-noyd-EK-to-me):   removal of ADENOIDS.

ADENOMA (ah-deh-NO-mah):   tumor of glandular cells. This is a benign (non-cancerous) tumor.

ADENOPATHY (ah-deh-NOP-ah-the):   condition of disease of glands. Often this refers to enlargement of glands.

ADNEXA UTERI (ad-NEKS-ah U-ter-i):   accessory structures of the uterus (ovaries and fallopian tubes).

ADRENAL GLANDS (ah-DRE-nal glanz):   two endocrine glands, each above a kidney. The adrenal glands produce hormones such as adrenalin (epinephrine) and cortisone.

ADRENALECTOMY (ah-dre-nal-EK-to-me):   removal (excision) of adrenal glands.

AIR SACS (ar saks):   thin-walled sacs within the lung. Inhaled oxygen passes into the blood from the sacs, and carbon dioxide passes out from the blood into the sacs to be exhaled.

ALBUMINURIA (al-bu-men-U-re-ah):   protein in the urine (an abnormal condition).

ALLERGIST (AL-er-jist):   medical doctor specializing in identifying and treating conditions of abnormal (excessive) sensitivity to foreign substances such as pollen, dust, foods, and drugs.

ALVEOLAR (al-VE-o-lar):   pertaining to air sacs (alveoli) within the lungs.

ALVEOLUS (al-ve-O-lus):   an air sac within the lung (pl. alveoli).

AMENORRHEA (a-men-o-RE-ah):   absence of menstrual periods.

AMNIOCENTESIS (am-ne-o-sen-TE-sis):   surgical puncture to remove fluid from the amnion (the sac surrounding the developing infant).

ANAL (A-nal):   pertaining to the anus (the opening of the digestive tract to the outside of the body).

ANALYSIS (ah-NAL-ih-sis):   breaking apart of a substance to understand its contents.

---

* No diacritical (accent) marks are used except ī to indicate the long i in words ending in -CYTE.

ANEMIA (ah-NE-me-ah): condition of less than normal numbers of red blood cells or amount of HEMOGLOBIN inside the red blood cells. Literally, anemia means lacking (AN-) in blood (-EMIA).

ANEMIC (ah-NE-mik): pertaining to anemia.

ANESTHESIOLOGIST (an-es-the-ze-OL-o-jist): medical doctor specializing in administering agents capable of bringing about loss of sensation and consciousness.

ANESTHESIOLOGY (an-es-the-ze-OL-o-je): study of how to administer agents capable of bringing about loss of sensation and consciousness.

ANGINA (an-JI-nah): sharp pain in the chest resulting from a decrease in blood supply to the heart muscle; also called angina pectoris (chest).

ANGIOGRAPHY (an-je-OG-rah-fe): process of recording (by x-ray) blood vessels after a dye is injected.

ANGIOPLASTY (AN-je-o-plas-te): surgical repair of a blood vessel. This term is most often used to describe a procedure in which a tube (catheter) is placed in a clogged artery and a balloon in the end of the tube is inflated to flatten the clogged material against the wall of the artery. This opens the blood vessel so that more blood can pass through.

ANOMALY (an-NOM-ah-le): an irregularity, anything that is not normal. See CONGENITAL ANOMALY.

ANTE MORTEM (AN-te MOR-tem): before death.

ANTE NATAL (AN-te NA-tal): before birth.

ANTE PARTUM (AN-te PAR-tum): before birth.

ANTERIOR (an-TE-re-or): located in the front (of the body or of a structure).

ANTIARRHYTHMIC (an-te-ah-RITH-mik): pertaining to a drug that works against or prevents abnormal heart beats (arrhythmias).

ANTIBIOTIC (an-tih-bi-OT-ik): pertaining to against (ANTI-) germ or bacterial life (BI/O). Antibiotics are made from primitive plants called molds.

ANTIBODY (AN-tih-bod-e): a substance that works against (ANTI-) germs ("bodies" of infection). Antibodies are produced by white blood cells when germs (antigens) enter the bloodstream.

ANTICOAGULANT (an-tih-ko-AG-u-lant): drug that prevents clotting (coagulation). Anticoagulants are given to a patient when there is danger of clots forming in blood vessels.

ANTIGEN (AN-tih-jen): a foreign agent that stimulates white blood cells to make antibodies. Antigens (such as bacteria and viruses) are then destroyed by the antibodies. This is known as an immune reaction.

ANTIHYPERTENSIVE (an-ti-hi-per-TEN-siv): a drug that reduces high blood pressure.

ANURIA (an-U-re-ah): condition of no urination.

ANUS (A-nus): opening of the rectum to the surface of the body; solid wastes (feces) leave the body through the anus.

AORTA (a-OR-tah): largest artery; it leads from the lower left chamber of the heart to arteries all over the body.

APNEA (AP-ne-ah): not (A-) able to breathe (PNEA).

APPENDECTOMY (ap-en-DEK-to-me):   removal of the appendix.

APPENDICITIS (ap-en-dih-SI-tis):   inflammation of the appendix.

APPENDIX (ah-PEN-dikz):   small sac that hangs from the beginning of the large intestine in the lower right area of the abdomen. It has no known digestive function.

AREOLA (ah-RE-o-lah):   dark, pigmented area around the nipple of the breast.

ARRHYTHMIA (a-RITH-me-ah):   abnormal heart rhythm.

ARTERIOLE (ar-TER-e-ol):   a small artery.

ARTERIOLITIS (ar-ter-e-o-LI-tis):   inflammation of small arteries.

ARTERIOSCLEROSIS (ar-ter-e-o-skle-RO-sis):   hardening of arteries. The most common form of arteriosclerosis is *atherosclerosis,* which is hardening of arteries caused by a collection of fatty, cholesterol-like deposits (plaque) in arteries.

ARTERY (AR-ter-e):   largest blood vessel. Arteries carry blood away from the heart.

ARTHRALGIA (ar-THRAL-je-ah):   pain in a joint.

ARTHRITIS (ar-THRI-tis):   inflammation in a joint.

ARTHROCENTESIS (ar-thro-sen-TE-sis):   surgical puncture to remove fluid from a joint.

ARTHROGRAM (AR-thro-gram):   x-ray record of a joint.

ARTHROPATHY (ar-THROP-ah-the):   disease of joints.

ARTHROSCOPE (AR-thro-skop):   an instrument to examine the inside of a joint.

ARTHROSCOPY (ar-THROS-ko-pe):   process of visual examination of a joint.

ARTHROSIS (ar-THRO-sis):   abnormal condition of a joint.

ASCITES (ah-SI-tez):   abnormal collection of fluid in the abdomen.

ASTHMA (AZ-mah):   difficult breathing caused by spasms of the bronchial tubes or swelling of their mucous membrane lining.

ATELECTASIS (ah-teh-LEK-tah-sis):   collapsed lung (ATEL- = "incomplete"; -ECTATASIS = "dilation").

ATHEROSCLEROSIS (ah-theh-ro-skle-RO-sis):   See ARTERIOSCLEROSIS.

ATRIUM (A-tre-um):   upper chamber of the heart (pl. atria).

ATROPHY (AT-ro-fe):   decrease in size of an organ.

AUDITORY CANAL (AW-dih-to-re kah-NAL):   passageway leading into the ear from the outside of the body.

AUDITORY NERVE (AW-dih-to-re nurv):   carries messages from the inner ear to the brain, making hearing possible.

AURA (AW-rah):   a peculiar sensation that comes before more definite signs of illness. An aura often precedes a migraine headache, warning the patient that an attack is beginning.

AUTOPSY (AW-top-se):   examination of a dead body to discover the actual cause of death; also called a post mortem exam or necropsy. Literally, the term means to see (-OPSY) with one's own (AUTO-) eyes.

AXILLARY (AKS-ih-lar-e):   pertaining to the armpit.

BALANITIS (bah-lah-NI-tis):   inflammation of the penis.

BARIUM (BAH-re-um):   a substance used as an opaque (x-rays can't pass through it) contrast medium for x-ray examination of the digestive tract.

BARIUM ENEMA (BAH-re-um EN-eh-mah): an x-ray picture of the lower digestive tract after injecting a solution of barium into the rectum.

BENIGN (be-NIN): not cancerous; a tumor that does not spread and is limited in growth.

BILATERAL (bi-LAT-er-al): pertaining to two (both) sides.

BILE (bil): a chemical that helps to break down and digest fats.

BILE DUCT (bil dukt): tube that carries BILE from the liver and gallbladder to the intestine.

BIOLOGY (bi-OL-o-je): study of life.

BIOPSY (BI-op-se): process of viewing living tissue. A sample of tissue is removed from an organ and then prepared for viewing under the microscope.

BLADDER (BLAD-der): see URINARY BLADDER.

BONE (bon): hard, rigid type of connective tissue that makes up most of the skeleton. It is composed of calcium salts.

BONE MARROW (bon MAH-ro): soft, sponge-like material in the inner part of bones. It is the place where blood cells are made.

BRADYCARDIA (bra-de-KAR-de-ah): condition of slow heartbeat.

BRAIN (bran): the organ in the head that controls the activities of the body.

BREAST (brest): one of two glands in the front of the chest that produce milk after childbirth.

BRONCHIAL TUBE (BRONG-ke-al tube): one of two tubes that carry air from the windpipe to the lungs. Also called a bronchus (pl. bronchi).

BRONCHIOLE (BRONG-ke-ol): small (-OLE) bronchial tube.

BRONCHITIS (brong-KI-tis): inflammation of the bronchial tubes.

BRONCHOSCOPE (BRONG-ko-skop): instrument to visually examine the bronchial tubes.

BRONCHOSCOPY (bron-KOS-ko-pe): visual examination of the bronchial tubes by passing an endoscope (bronchoscope) through the trachea (windpipe) into the bronchi.

BRONCHUS (BRONG-kus) pl. BRONCHI (BRON-chi): see BRONCHIAL TUBE.

CALCANEUS (kal-KA-ne-us): heel bone.

CALCULUS (KAL-ku-lus): a stone.

CAPILLAROPATHY (kap-ih-lar-OP-ah-the): disease of capillaries.

CAPILLARY (KAP-ih-lar-e): smallest blood vessel (pl. capillaries).

CARCINOMA (kar-sih-NO-mah): cancerous tumor. Carcinomas form from epithelial cells, which line the internal organs as well as cover the outside of the body.

CARDIAC (KAR-de-ak): pertaining to the heart.

CARDIOLOGIST (kar-de-OL-o-jist): specialist in the study of the heart and heart disorders.

CARDIOLOGY (kar-de-OL-o-je): study of the heart.

CARDIOMEGALY (kar-de-o-MEG-ah-le): enlargement of the heart.

CARDIOMYOPATHY (kar-de-o-mi-OP-ah-the): disease of heart muscle.

CARDIOVASCULAR SURGEON (kar-de-o-VAS-ku-lar SUR-jin): doctor specializing in operating on the heart and blood vessels.

CARPALS (KAR-palz):   wrist bones.

CARTILAGE (KAR-tih-lij):   flexible, fibrous connective tissue, found attached to bones and at the ends of bones at the joints. It is more flexible than bone and firmer than muscle.

CATARACT (KAT-ah-rakt):   clouding of the lens of the eye.

CAT SCAN (kat scan):   computerized axial tomography. See CT SCAN.

CELL (sel):   the smallest unit or part of an organ.

CELLULITIS (sel-u-LI-tis):   inflammation of soft tissue under the skin; marked by swelling, redness, and pain and caused by bacterial infection.

CEPHALGIA (seh-FAL-je-ah):   pain within the head (headache). Cephalgia is a shortened form of *cephalalgia.*

CEPHALIC (seh-FAL-ik):   pertaining to the head.

CEREBELLAR (ser-eh-BEL-ar):   pertaining to the cerebellum; the lower, back part of the brain.

CEREBELLUM (ser-eh-BEL-um):   lower, back part of the brain which coordinates muscle movement and balance.

CEREBRAL (seh-RE-bral or SER-e-bral):   pertaining to the cerebrum, the largest part of the brain.

CEREBROVASCULAR ACCIDENT (seh-re-bro-VAS-ku-lar AK-sih-dent):   a disorder of blood vessels within the cerebrum. A CVA results from poor blood supply to the brain. Also called a STROKE.

CEREBRUM (seh-RE-brum):   largest part of the brain. The cerebrum controls many functions including speech, hearing, vision, thought, reasoning, and body movements.

CERVICAL (SER-vih-kal):   pertaining to the neck of the body or the neck of the uterus (cervix).

CERVICAL REGION (SER-vih-kal RE-jin):   the seven backbones in the area of the neck.

CERVICAL VERTEBRA (SER-vih-kal VER-teh-brah):   a backbone in the neck.

CERVIX (SER-viks):   the lower, neck-like portion of the uterus (womb) that opens into the vagina.

CESAREAN SECTION (se-SA-re-an SEK-shun):   incision of the uterus to remove the fetus at birth.

CHEMOTHERAPY (ke-mo-THER-ah-pe):   treatment with drugs; most often used to refer to drug treatment for cancer.

CHOLECYSTECTOMY (ko-le-sis-TEK-to-me):   removal of the gallbladder.

CHOLEDOCHOTOMY (ko-led-o-KOT-o-me):   incision of the common bile duct.

CHOLELITHIASIS (ko-le-lih-THI-ah-sis):   abnormal condition of gallstones.

CHONDROMA (kon-DRO-mah):   tumor (benign) of cartilage.

CHRONIC (KRON-ik):   lasting over a long period of time (CHRON/O).

CIRCULATORY SYSTEM (SER-ku-lah-tor-e SIS-tem):   the organs (heart and blood vessels) that carry blood throughout the body. This system also includes the vessels that carry lymph (a clear fluid containing white blood cells) within the body.

CIRRHOSIS (seh-RO-sis): liver disease with deterioration of liver cells; often caused by alcoholism and poor nutrition.

CLAVICLE (KLAV-ih-kuhl): collar bone.

CLINICAL (KLIN-eh-kal): pertaining to the bedside or clinic. Clinical work involves patient care.

COCCYGEAL (kok-sih-JE-al): pertaining to the tailbone (coccyx).

COCCYGEAL REGION (kok-sih-JE-al RE-jin): the four fused (joined together) bones at the base of the spinal column (backbone).

COCCYX (KOK-siks): tailbone.

COLITIS (ko-LI-tis): inflammation of the colon (large intestine).

COLON (KO-lon): large intestine (bowel).

COLONOSCOPY (ko-lon-OS-ko-pe): visual examination of the colon.

COLORECTAL SURGEON (ko-lo-REK-tal SUR-jin): doctor specializing in operating on the colon and rectum (lower part of the gastrointestinal tract).

COLOSTOMY (ko-LOS-to-me): opening of the colon to the outside of the body.

CONGENITAL (kon-JEN-ih-tal): pertaining to conditions that are present at birth, regardless of their causes.

CONGENITAL ANOMALY (con-JEN-ih-tal ah -NOM-ah-le): an irregularity or abnormality that is present at birth.

CONIZATION (ko-nih-ZA-shun): removal of a wedge-shaped piece (cone) of tissue from the cervix as diagnosis and treatment of early cancer of the cervix.

CONJUNCTIVA (kon-junk-TI-vah): thin protective membrane over the front of the eye and attached to the eyelids.

CONJUNCTIVITIS (kon-junk-ti-VI-tis): inflammation of the conjunctiva.

CONNECTIVE TISSUE (kon-NEK-tiv TIS-u): fibrous tissue that supports and connects internal organs, bones, and walls of blood vessels.

CORIUM (KOR-e-um): middle layer of the skin below the epidermis; also called DERMIS.

CORNEA (KOR-ne-ah): transparent layer over the front of the eye. It bends light so that it is focused on sensitive cells in the back of the eye.

CORONAL PLANE (kor-O-nal plan): see FRONTAL PLANE.

CORONARY (KOR-on-ary): pertaining to the heart. *Coronary arteries* branch from the aorta (largest artery) to bring oxygen-rich blood to the heart muscle.

COSTOCHONDRAL (kos-to-KON-dral): pertaining to a rib and its cartilage.

CRANIAL CAVITY (KRA-ne-al KAV-ih-te): the space surrounded by the skull which contains the brain and other organs.

CRANIOTOMY (kra-ne-OT-o-me): incision of the skull.

CRANIUM (KRA-ne-um): skull.

CREATININE (kre-AT-tih-nin): nitrogen-containing waste that is removed from the blood by the kidney and excreted in urine.

CRYPTORCHISM (kript-OR-kism): condition of undescended (CRYPT- means "hidden") testis. The testis is not in the scrotal sac at birth.

CT SCAN: computerized tomography. A series of x-ray pictures that show the body in cross-section (transverse view), as if to divide the body into an upper and lower portion. Also called a CAT SCAN.

CYSTITIS (sis-TI-tis):   inflammation of the urinary bladder.

CYSTOSCOPE (SIS-to-skop):   instrument (endoscope) to view the urinary bladder.

CYSTOSCOPY (sis-TOS-ko-pe):   process of viewing the urinary bladder using a cystoscope.

CYTOLOGY (si-TOL-o-je):   study of cells.

DEBRIDEMENT (de-BRED-ment):   removal of diseased tissue from the skin.

DERMATITIS (der-mah-TI-tis):   inflammation of the skin.

DERMATOLOGIST (der-mah-TOL-o-jist):   specialist in treatment of the skin and skin diseases.

DERMATOLOGY (der-mah-TOL-o-je):   study of the skin.

DERMATOSIS (der-mah-TO-sis):   abnormal condition of the skin.

DERMIS (DER-mis):   middle layer of the skin, below the epidermis; corium.

DIABETES MELLITUS (di-ah-BE-tez MEL-li-tus):   abnormal condition marked by deficient insulin (hormone from the pancreas) in the blood. This deficiency causes sugar to remain in the blood instead of entering the cells of the body. Called diabetes, from a Greek word meaning a "siphon," through which water passes easily; one symptom of diabetes is frequent urination.

DIAGNOSIS (di-ag-NO-sis):   complete (DIA-) knowledge (-GNOSIS) about the patient's condition.

DIALYSIS (di-AL-ih-sis):   complete (DIA-) separation (-LYSIS) of the wastes (urea) from the blood when the kidneys have failed. See also HEMODIALYSIS and PERITONEAL DIALYSIS.

DIAPHRAGM (DI-ah-fram):   the muscle that separates the chest from the abdomen.

DIARRHEA (di-ar-RE-ah):   flow (-RRHEA) through (DIA-). This is the discharge of watery wastes from the end of the digestive tract.

DIGESTIVE SYSTEM (di-JES-tiv SIS-tem):   the organs that bring food into the body and break it down so that it can enter the bloodstream. Food that cannot be broken down is removed from the body through the rectum and anus (end of the digestive system).

DILATION (di-LA-shun):   widening, dilatation.

DILATION AND CURETTAGE (di-LA-shun and kur-eh-TAJ):   widening of the opening of the cervix and scraping (curettage) the inner lining of the uterus; D & C.

DISK: piece of cartilage that is between each backbone.

DIURETICS (di-u-RET-iks):   drugs that cause the kidneys to allow more fluid to leave the body; used to treat high blood pressure. DI- (from DIA-) means "complete" and UR- means "urine."

DIVERTICULOSIS (di-ver-tik-u-LO-sis):   abnormal condition of small pouches or sacs in the lining of the intestine.

DUODENUM (du-o-DE-num):   first part of the small intestine.

DYSMENORRHEA (dis-men-o-RE-ah):   painful menstrual flow.

DYSPEPSIA (dis-PEP-se-ah):   condition of painful (DYS-) digestion (-PEPSIA).

DYSPHAGIA (dis-FA-je-ah):   difficult, painful swallowing.

DYSPLASIA (dis-PLA-se-ah):   abnormality in formation (-PLASIA) of cells. This means that normal cells change in size, shape, and organization.

DYSPNEA (DISP-ne-ah):   painful, difficult, breathing (-PNEA).

DYSURIA (dis-U-re-ah):   painful (DYS-) urination (-URIA).

EAR (ear):   organ that receives sound waves and transmits them to nerves leading to the brain.

EARDRUM (EAR-drum):   membrane that separates the outer and inner parts of the ear; tympanic membrane.

ECTOPIC PREGNANCY (ek-TOP-ik PREG-nan-se):   a pregnancy that is not in the uterus. The most common place for an ectopic pregnancy to occur is in the fallopian tubes.

EDEMA (eh-DE-mah):   Swelling in tissues; often caused by retention (holding back) of fluid and salt by the kidneys.

ELECTROCARDIOGRAM (e-lek-tro-KAR-de-o-gram):   record of the electricity in the heart.

ELECTROENCEPHALOGRAM (e-lek-tro-en-SEF-ah-lo-gram):   record of the electricity in the brain.

ELECTROENCEPHALOGRAPHY (e-lek-tro-en-sef-ah-LOG-rah-fe):   process of recording the electricity in the brain.

EMBRYO (EM-bre-o):   a new organism in the earliest stage of development. After the second month the unborn baby is called a fetus.

EMERGENCY MEDICINE (e-MER-jen-se MED-ih-sin):   care of patients that requires sudden and immediate action.

ENCEPHALITIS (en-sef-al-LI-tis):   inflammation of the brain.

ENCEPHALOPATHY (en-sef-ah-LOP-ah-the):   disease of the brain.

ENDOCRINE GLANDS (EN-do-krin glanz):   organs that produce hormones. Hormones enter the blood and travel to other organs and glands, causing an increase or decrease in their ability to function.

ENDOCRINE SYSTEM (EN-do-krin SIS-tem):   the endocrine glands. The pituitary, thyroid, testes, ovaries, pancreas, and adrenal glands are part of the endocrine system.

ENDOCRINOLOGIST (en-do-krih-NOL-o-jist):   specialist in the study of endocrine glands and their disorders.

ENDOCRINOLOGY (en-do-krih-NOL-o-je):   study of the endocrine glands.

ENDOMETRIUM (en-do-ME-tre-um):   inner lining of the uterus.

ENDOSCOPE (EN-do-skop):   instrument to view a hollow organ or body cavity. It is a hollow metal or fiber tube fitted with a lens system that allows viewing in several directions. It has a light source, power cord, and power source.

ENDOSCOPY (en-DOS-ko-pe):   process of viewing the inside of the body (hollow organs or body cavities) by using an endoscope (the instrument used to perform endoscopy).

ENTERITIS (en-teh-RI-tis):   inflammation of the small intestine.

EPIDERMIS (ep-i-DER-mis):   the outer (EPI-) layer of the skin (-DERMIS).

EPIDURAL HEMATOMA (ep-ih-DUR-al he-mah-TO-mah):   mass of blood above the dura mater, which is the outermost layer of the membranes surrounding the brain and spinal cord.

EPIGLOTTIS (ep-ih-GLOT-tis): flap of cartilage that covers the mouth of the windpipe when swallowing occurs, so that food does not enter the windpipe.

EPIGLOTTITIS (ep-ih-glo-TI-tis): inflammation of the epiglottis.

EPITHELIAL (ep-ih-THE-le-al): pertaining to skin cells. This term originally described the cells upon (EPI-) the nipple (THELI-) of the breast. Now, it refers to all cells lining the inner part of internal organs as well as covering the outside of the body.

ERYTHROCYTE (e-RITH-ro-sīt): red blood cell.

ERYTHROCYTOSIS (e-rith-ro-sī-TO-sis): abnormal condition (slight increase in numbers) of red blood cells.

ERYTHROMYCIN (e-rith-ro-MI-sin): an antibiotic that is produced from a red (ERYTHR/O) mold (-MYCIN).

ESOPHAGEAL (e-sof-ah-JE-al): pertaining to the esophagus.

ESOPHAGITIS (e-sof-ah-JI-tis): inflammation of the esophagus.

ESOPHAGUS (e-SOF-ah-gus): tube that carries food from the throat to the stomach.

EUSTACHIAN TUBE (u-STA-she-an tub): channel that connects the middle part of the ear with the throat.

EXCISION (ek-SIZH-un): to cut out; remove; resect.

EXOCRINE GLANDS (EK-so-krin glanz): glands that produce (secrete) chemicals that leave the body through tubes or ducts. Examples of exocrine glands are tear, sweat, and salivary glands.

EXOPHTHALMOS (ek-sof-THAL-mos): abnormal condition of eyeball protrusion. This is often associated with oversecretion of hormone from the thyroid gland (hyperthyroidism).

EXTRAHEPATIC (eks-tra-heh-PAT-ik): pertaining to outside the liver.

EXTRAPULMONARY (eks-trah-PUL-mo-nah-re): outside the lungs.

EYE (i): organ that receives light waves and transmits them to the brain.

FALLOPIAN TUBES (fah-LO-pe-an tubz): two tubes that lead from the ovaries to the uterus. They transport the egg cell to the uterus; also called *uterine tubes.*

FAMILY MEDICINE (FAM-ih-le MED-ih-sin): primary care of all members of the family on a continuing basis.

FELLOWSHIP TRAINING (FEL-o-ship TRA-ning): postgraduate training for doctors in specialized fields. The training can include clinical (patient care) and research (laboratory) work.

FEMALE REPRODUCTIVE SYSTEM (FE-mal re-pro-DUK-tiv SIS-tem): organs that produce and transport egg cells and secrete female hormones, such as estrogen and progesterone. The system also contains an organ (uterus) that permits the growth of the embryo and fetus.

FEMUR (FE-mer): thigh bone.

FETUS (FE-tus): the unborn infant after the second month of pregnancy.

FIBROIDS (FI-broydz): benign growths of muscle tissue in the uterus.

FIBULA (FIB-u-lah):   smaller lower leg bone.

FIXATION (fik-SA-shun):   the act of holding, sewing, or fastening a part in a fixed position.

FRACTURE (FRAK-tur):   breaking of a bone.

FRONTAL (FRUN-tal):   pertaining to the front; anterior.

FRONTAL PLANE (FRUN-tal plan):   an imaginary line that divides an organ or the body into a front and back portion. Also called coronal plane.

FRONTAL SECTION (FRUN-tal SEK-shun):   a cut (section) through the body that divides it into front and back parts.

GALLBLADDER (GAL-bla-der):   sac below the liver that stores bile and delivers it to the small intestine.

GASTRECTOMY (gas-TREK-to-me):   excision (removal) of the stomach.

GASTRIC (GAS-trik):   pertaining to the stomach.

GASTRITIS (gas-TRI-tis):   inflammation of the stomach.

GASTROENTERITIS (gas-tro-en-teh-RI-tis):   inflammation of the stomach and the intestines.

GASTROENTEROLOGIST (gas-tro-en-ter-OL-o-jist):   specialist in treatment of stomach and intestinal disorders.

GASTROENTEROLOGY (gas-tro-en-ter-OL-o-je):   study of the stomach and intestines.

GASTROSCOPE (GAS-tro-skop):   instrument used to view the stomach. It is passed down the throat and esophagus into the stomach.

GASTROSCOPY (gas-TROS-ko-pe):   visual examination of the stomach with an endoscope.

GASTROTOMY (gas-TROT-o-me):   incision of the stomach.

GERIATRICIAN (jer-e-ah-TRI-shun):   specialist in the treatment of diseases of old age.

GERIATRICS (jer-e-AH-triks):   treatment of disorders of old age.

GLAND (gland):   a group of cells that secrete (send) chemicals to the outside of the body (EXOCRINE GLANDS) or directly into the bloodstream (ENDOCRINE GLANDS).

GLAUCOMA (glaw-KO-mah):   increase of fluid pressure within the eye; fluid is formed more rapidly than it is removed. The increased pressure damages the sensitive cells in the back of the eye and vision is disturbed.

GLYCOSURIA (gli-ko-SU-re-ah):   abnormal condition of sugar in the urine.

GOITER (GOY-ter):   enlargement of the thyroid gland.

GRAVES' DISEASE (gravs dih-ZEZ):   see HYPERTHYROIDISM.

GYNECOLOGIST (gi-neh-KOL-o-jist):   specialist in medical and surgical treatment of female disorders.

GYNECOLOGY (gi-neh-KOL-o-je):   study of female disorders.

HAIR FOLLICLE (hahr FOL-ih-kl):   a pouch-like depression in the skin in which a hair develops.

HAIR ROOT (hahr rut):   that part of the hair from which growth occurs.

HEART (hart):   hollow, muscular organ in the chest that pumps blood throughout the body.

HEMATEMESIS (he-mah-TEM-eh-sis):   vomiting (-EMESIS) blood (HEMAT-).

HEMATOLOGIST (he-mah-TOL-o-jist):   specialist in blood and blood disorders.

HEMATOMA (he-mah-TO-mah):   mass or collection of blood under the skin; commonly called a bruise or black-and-blue mark.

HEMATURIA (he-mah-TUR-e-ah):   abnormal condition of blood in the urine.

HEMODIALYSIS (he-mo-di-AL-i-sis):   use of a kidney machine to filter blood to remove waste materials, such as urea. Blood leaves the body, enters the machine, and is carried back to the body through a catheter (tube).

HEMOGLOBIN (HE-mo-glo-bin):   protein found in red blood cells. Hemoglobin combines with oxygen and carries it in the blood.

HEMORRHAGE (HEM-or-ij):   bursting forth of blood.

HEPATIC (heh-PAT-ik):   pertaining to the liver.

HEPATITIS (hep-ah-TI-tis):   inflammation of the liver.

HEPATOMA (hep-ah-TO-mah):   tumor of the liver.

HEPATOMEGALY (hep-ah-to-MEG-ah-le):   enlargement of the liver.

HERNIA (HER-ne-ah):   bulge or protrusion of an organ or part of an organ through the wall of the cavity that usually contains it. In an inguinal hernia, part of the wall of the abdomen weakens and the intestine bulges out or into the scrotal sac (in males).

HIATAL HERNIA (hi-A-tal HER-ne-ah):   upward protrusion of the wall of the stomach into the lower part of the esophagus.

HODGKIN'S DISEASE (HOJ-kinz di-ZEZ):   malignant (cancerous) tumor of lymph nodes.

HORMONE (HOR-mon):   chemical made by a gland, sent directly into the bloodstream and not to the outside of the body. Glands that produce hormones are called ENDOCRINE GLANDS.

HUMERUS (HU-mer-us):   upper arm bone.

HYPERGLYCEMIA (hi-per-gli-SE-me-ah):   higher than normal levels of sugar in the blood.

HYPERPARATHYROIDISM (hi-per-par-ah-THI-royd-ism):   higher than normal levels of parathyroid hormone in the blood.

HYPERTENSION (hi-per-TEN-shun):   high blood pressure.

HYPERTHYROIDISM (hi-per-THI-royd-izm):   excessive activity of the thyroid gland. Also known as *Graves' disease.*

HYPERTROPHY (hi-PER-tro-fe):   enlargement or overgrowth of an organ or part due to an increase in size of individual cells.

HYPODERMIC (hi-po-DER-mik):   pertaining to under or below the skin.

HYPOGLYCEMIA (hi-po-gli-SE-me-ah):   lower than normal levels of sugar in the blood.

HYPOPHYSEAL (hi-po-FIZ-e-al):   pertaining to the pituitary gland.

HYPOPITUITARISM (hi-po-pi-TU-i-tah-rizm):   decrease or stoppage of function of the pituitary gland.

HYPOTENSIVE (hi-po-TEN-siv):   pertaining to low blood pressure, or to a person with abnormally low blood pressure.

HYPOTHYROIDISM (hi-po-THI-royd-izm):   lower than normal activity of the thyroid gland.

HYSTERECTOMY (his-teh-REK-to-me):   excision (removal) of the uterus, either through the abdominal wall (abdominal hysterectomy) or through the vagina (vaginal hysterectomy). A total hysterectomy is removal of the entire uterus, including the cervix.

IATROGENIC (i-ah-tro-JEN-ik):   pertaining to an abnormal condition in a patient that results unexpectedly from a specific treatment.

ILEUM (IL-e-um):   third part of the small intestine.

ILIUM (IL-e-um):   high side portion of the hip bone.

INCISION (in-SIZH-un):   cutting into the body or an organ.

INFARCTION (in-FARK-shun):   area of dead tissue caused by decreased blood flow to that part of the body.

INFECTIOUS DISEASE SPECIALIST (in-FEK-shus dih-ZEZ SPESH-ah-list):   specialist in treating disorders that are caused and spread by microorganisms such as bacteria and viruses.

INFILTRATE (IN-fil-trat):   material that accumulates in an organ; often used to describe a solid material and fluid collection in the lung.

INGUINAL (ING-gwi-nal):   pertaining to the groin; the area where the legs are joined to the body.

INSULIN (IN-su-lin):   endocrine hormone produced by the pancreas and released into the bloodstream. Insulin allows sugar to leave the blood and enter body cells.

INTERNAL MEDICINE (in-TER-nal MED-ih-sin):   branch of medicine specializing in the diagnosis of disorders and treatment with drugs.

INTERVERTEBRAL (in-ter-VER-teh-bral):   pertaining to lying between two backbones. A disk is an intervertebral structure.

INTRA-ABDOMINAL (in-trah-ab-DOM-ih-nal):   pertaining to within the abdomen.

INTRAUTERINE (in-trah-U-ter-in):   pertaining to within the uterus.

INTRAVENOUS (in-trah-VE-nus):   pertaining to within a vein.

INTRAVENOUS PYELOGRAM (in-trah-VEN-nus PI-eh-lo-gram):   x-ray record of the kidney after dye is injected into a vein. PYEL/O means "renal pelvis," the central section of the kidney.

IRIS (I-ris):   colored (pigmented) portion of the eye.

ISCHEMIA (is-KE-me-ah):   deficiency of blood flow to a part of the body, caused by narrowing or obstruction of a blood vessel.

JAUNDICE (JAWN-dis):   orange-yellow coloration of the skin and other tissues. This symptom may be caused by accumulation of a pigment (bilirubin) in the blood when the diseased liver is not able to remove bile (containing bilirubin) from the body.

JEJUNUM (jeh-JU-num):   second part of the small intestine.

JOINT (joynt): space where two or more bones come together.

KIDNEY (KID-ne): organ behind the abdomen that makes urine by filtering wastes from the blood.

LAPAROSCOPY (lap-ah-ROS-ko-pe): visual examination of the abdomen (LAPAR/O). A small incision is made near the navel, and an instrument is inserted to view abdominal organs.

LAPAROTOMY (lap-ah-ROT-o-me): incision of the abdomen. A large incision is made across the abdomen, and the abdomen is opened to examine its organs.

LARGE INTESTINE (larj in-TES-tin): part of the intestine that receives undigested material from the small intestine and transports it to the outside of the body; colon.

LARYNGEAL (lah-rin-JE-al): pertaining to the larynx (voice box).

LARYNGECTOMY (lah-rin-JEK-to-me): removal of the larynx (voice box).

LARYNGITIS (lah-rin-JI-tis): inflammation of the larynx.

LARYNGOTRACHEITIS (lah-ring-go-tra-ke-I-tis): inflammation of the larynx and the trachea (windpipe).

LARYNX (LAR-inks): voice box; located at the top of the trachea (windpipe) and containing the vocal cords.

LATERAL (LAT-er-al): pertaining to the side.

LENS (lenz): the structure behind the pupil of the eye that bends light rays so that they are properly beamed at the retina in the back of the eye.

LESION (LE-zhun): any damage to a part of the body, caused by disease or trauma.

LEUKEMIA (lu-KE-me-ah): malignant (cancerous) condition of excess numbers of white blood cells (leukocytes) in the blood and bone marrow.

LEUKOCYTE (LU-ko-sīt): white blood cell.

LIGAMENT (LIG-ah-ment): connective tissue that joins bones to other bones.

LITHOTRIPSY (lith-o-TRIP-se): process of crushing (-TRIPSY) a stone in the urinary tract using ultrasonic vibrations.

LIVER (LIV-er): organ in the upper right region of the abdomen that makes BILE, stores sugar, and produces proteins to help blood clot.

LOBE (lob): part of an organ, especially of the brain, lungs, or glands.

LUMBAR (LUM-bar): pertaining to the loins, the part of the back between the chest and the hip.

LUMBAR REGION (LUM-bar RE-jin): pertaining to the backbones that lie between the thoracic (chest) and sacral (lower back) regions.

LUMBAR VERTEBRA (LUM-bar VER-teh-brah): a backbone in the region between the chest and the lower back.

LUNG (lung): one of the two paired organs in the chest through which oxygen enters and carbon dioxide leaves the body.

LUNG CAPILLARIES (lung KAP-ih-lar-ez): tiny blood vessels surrounding lung tissue and through which gases pass into and out of the bloodstream.

LYMPH (limf): clear fluid that is found in lymph vessels and produced from fluid surrounding cells. Lymph contains white blood cells (lymphocytes) that fight disease.

LYMPH NODE (limf nod): stationary collection of lymph cells. Lymph nodes are found all over the body.

LYMPHADENOPATHY (lim-fad-e-NOP-ah-the): disease of lymph nodes.

LYMPHANGIOGRAM (lim-FAN-je-o-gram): x-ray record of lymph vessels after dye is injected into soft tissue of the foot.

LYMPHANGIOGRAPHY (lim-fan-je-OG-rah-fe): process of recording (by x-ray) lymph vessels after dye is injected into soft tissue of the foot.

LYMPHATIC VESSELS (lim-FAT-ik VES-elz): tubes that carry lymph from tissues to the bloodstream (into a vein in the neck region); lymph vessels.

LYMPHOCYTE (LIMF-o-sīt): white blood cell that is found within lymph and lymph nodes.

MAGNETIC RESONANCE IMAGING (mag-NET-ik REZ-o-nans IM-aj-ing): picture of the body using magnetic waves. Organs can be seen in three planes: frontal (front to back), sagittal (side to side), and transverse (cross-section).

MALE REPRODUCTIVE SYSTEM (mal re-pro-DUK-tiv SIS-tem): organs that produce sperm cells and male hormones, such as testosterone.

MALIGNANT (mah-LIG-nant): tending to become progressively worse; used to describe cancerous tumors that invade and spread to distant organs.

MAMMARY (MAM-er-e): pertaining to the breast.

MAMMOGRAM (MAM-o-gram): x-ray record of the breast.

MAMMOGRAPHY (mam-OG-rah-fe): process of x-ray recording of the breast.

MAMMOPLASTY (MAM-o-plas-te): surgical repair (reconstruction) of the breast.

MASTECTOMY (mas-TEK-to-me): removal (excision) of the breast.

MEDIASTINAL (me-de-ah-STI-nal): pertaining to the MEDIASTINUM.

MEDIASTINUM (me-de-ah-STI-num): space between the lungs in the chest. It contains the heart, large blood vessels, trachea, esophagus, thymus gland, and lymph nodes.

MEDULLA OBLONGATA (meh-DUL-ah ob-lon-GOT-ah): lower part of the brain, near the spinal cord. It controls breathing and heart function.

MENINGITIS (men-in-JI-tis): inflammation of the meninges (the membranes around the brain and spinal cord).

MENORRHAGIA (men-o-RA-je-ah): excessive bleeding from the uterus during the time of menstruation.

MENORRHEA (men-o-RE-ah): normal discharge of blood and tissue from the uterine lining during menstruation.

MENSES (MEN-sez): menstruation; menstrual period.

MENSTRUATION (men-stru-A-shun): breakdown of the lining of the uterus that occurs every four weeks during the active reproductive period of the female.

METACARPALS (met-ah-KAR-palz): bones of the hand between the wrist bones (carpals) and the finger bones (phalanges).

METASTASIS (meh-TAS-tah-sis): spread of a cancerous tumor to a distant organ or location; literally means beyond (META-) control (-STASIS).

METATARSALS (meh-tah-TAR-sels): foot bones.

MIGRAINE (MI-gran): attacks of headache, usually on one side of the head, caused by changes in blood vessel size and accompanied by nausea, vomiting, and sensitivity to light (photophobia). From the French word *migraine,* meaning "severe head pain."

MOUTH (mowth): the opening that forms the beginning of the digestive system.

MRI: see MAGNETIC RESONANCE IMAGING.

MUSCLE (MUS-el): connective tissue that contracts to make movement possible.

MUSCULAR (MUS-ku-lar): pertaining to muscles.

MUSCULOSKELETAL SYSTEM (mus-ku-lo-SKEL-e-tal SIS-tem): organs that support the body and allow it to move. These include muscles, bones, joints, and connective tissues such as tendons and ligaments.

MYALGIA (mi-AL-je-ah): pain in a muscle or muscles.

MYELOGRAM (MI-eh-lo-gram): x-ray record of the spinal cord.

MYOCARDIAL (mi-o-KAR-de-al): pertaining to the muscle of the heart.

MYOCARDIAL INFARCTION (mi-o-KAR-de-al in-FARK-shun): area of dead tissue in heart muscle; also known as a heart attack or an MI.

MYOMA (mi-O-mah): tumor (benign) of muscle.

MYOSARCOMA (mi-o-sar-KO-mah): tumor (malignant) of muscle. SARC- means "flesh," indicating that the tumor is of connective tissue origin.

MYOSITIS (mi-o-SI-tis): inflammation of a muscle.

MYRINGOTOMY (mir-in-GOT-o-me): incision of the eardrum.

NASAL (NA-zel): pertaining to the nose.

NAUSEA (NAW-se-ah): an unpleasant sensation in the upper abdomen, often leading to vomiting. The term comes from the Greek *nausia,* meaning "sea sickness."

NECROSIS (neh-KRO-sis): death of cells.

NEONATAL (ne-o-NA-tal): pertaining to new birth; the period of first four weeks after birth.

NEOPLASM (NE-o-plazm): any new growth of tissue; a tumor.

NEOPLASTIC (ne-o-PLAS-tik): pertaining to a new growth or neoplasm.

NEPHRECTOMY (neh-FREK-to-me): removal (excision) of a kidney.

NEPHRITIS (neh-FRI-tis): inflammation of the kidneys.

NEPHROLOGIST (neh-FROL-o-jist): specialist in diagnosis and treatment of kidney diseases.

NEPHROLOGY (neh-FROL-o-je): study of the kidney and its diseases.

NEPHROPATHY (neh-FROP-ah-the): disease of the kidney.

NEPHROSIS (neh-FRO-sis): abnormal condition of the kidney. This condition is often associated with a deterioration of kidney tubules.

NEPHROSTOMY (neh-FROS-to-me): opening from the kidney to the outside of the body.

NERVOUS SYSTEM (NER-vus SIS-tem): organs (brain, spinal cord, and nerves) that transmit electrical messages throughout the body.

NEURAL (NU-ral): pertaining to nerves.

NEURALGIA (nu-RAL-je-ah):   nerve pain.

NEURITIS (nu-RI-tis):   inflammation of a nerve.

NEUROLOGIST (nu-ROL-o-jist):   specialist in the diagnosis and treatment of nerve disorders.

NEUROLOGY (nu-ROL-o-je):   study of the nervous system and nerve disorders.

NEUROSURGEON (nu-ro-SUR-jin):   doctor who operates on the organs of the nervous system (brain, spinal cord, and nerves).

NEUROTOMY (nu-ROT-o-me):   incision (cutting) of a nerve.

NEVUS (NE-vus):   pigmented lesion on the skin; a mole.

NOCTURIA (nok-TU-re-ah):   excessive urination at night (NOCT/O)

NOSE (noz):   the structure that is the organ of smell and permits air to enter the body.

OBSTETRIC (ob-STEH-trik):   pertaining to pregnancy, labor, and the delivery of an infant.

OBSTETRICIAN (ob-steh-TRISH-un):   specialist in the delivery of a baby and care of the mother during pregnancy and labor.

OBSTETRICS (ob-STET-riks):   branch of surgery that deals with pregnancy, labor, and delivery of an infant. The Latin word *obstetrix* means "midwife."

OCULAR (OK-u-lar):   pertaining to the eye.

ONCOGENIC (ong-ko-JEN-ik):   pertaining to producing (GEN) tumors.

ONCOLOGICAL (ong-ko-LOG-ih-kal):   pertaining to the study of tumors.

ONCOLOGIST (ong-KOL-o-jist):   medical doctor who specializes in the study and treatment of tumors.

ONCOLOGY (ong-KOL-o-je):   study of tumors.

OOPHORECTOMY (o-off-o-REK-to-me):   removal (excision) of an ovary or ovaries.

OOPHORITIS (o-off-o-RI-tis):   inflammation of an ovary.

OPHTHALMOLOGIST (off-thal-MOL-o-jist):   specialist in the study of the eye and treatment of eye disorders.

OPHTHALMOLOGY (off-thal-MOL-o-je):   study of the eye; diagnosis and treatment of eye disorders.

OPHTHALMOSCOPE (off-THAL-mo-skop):   instrument to visually examine the eye.

OPTIC NERVE (OP-tik nerv):   nerve in the back of the eye that transmits light waves to the brain.

OPTICIAN (op-TISH-an):   specialist in providing eye glasses by filling prescriptions.

OPTOMETRIST (op-TOM-eh-trist):   specialist trained to examine and test eyes and prescribe corrective lenses.

ORAL (OR-al):   pertaining to the mouth.

ORCHIDECTOMY (or-kih-DEK-to-me):   removal (excision) of a testicle; orchiectomy.

ORCHIOPEXY (or-ke-o-PEK-se):   surgical fixation of the testicle (testis) into its proper location within the scrotum. This surgery corrects CRYPTORCHISM.

ORCHITIS (or-KI-tis):   inflammation of a testicle.

ORGAN (OR-gan):   an independent part of the body, composed of different tissues working together to do a specific job.

ORTHOPEDIST (or-tho-PE-dist):   specialist in surgical correction of musculoskeletal (muscles, bones, and joints) disorders. This doctor was originally concerned with straightening (ORTH/O) bones in the legs of deformed children (PED).

OSTEITIS (os-te-I-tis):   inflammation of a bone.

OSTEOARTHRITIS (os-te-o-ar-THRI-tis):   inflammation of bones and joints. This is a disease of older people, marked by stiffness and pain and degeneration of joints.

OSTEOMA (os-te-O-mah):   tumor (benign) of bone.

OSTEOMYELITIS (os-te-o-mi-eh-LI-tis):   inflammation of bone and bone marrow (MYEL-). This condition is caused by a bacterial infection.

OTALGIA (o-TAL-je-ah):   pain in the ear.

OTITIS (o-TI-tis):   inflammation of the ear.

OTOLARYNGOLOGIST (o-to-lar-in-GOL-o-jist):   specialist in treatment of diseases of the ear, nose, and throat.

OVARIAN (o-VA-re-an):   pertaining to an ovary or ovaries.

OVARY (O-vah-re):   one of two organs in the female abdomen that produces egg cells and female hormones.

PANCREAS (PAN-kre-us):   gland that produces digestive juices that work on food in the small intestine, and the hormone INSULIN.

PANCREATECTOMY (pan-kre-ah-TEK-to-me):   removal (excision) of the pancreas.

PANCREATITIS (pan-kre-ah-TI-tis):   inflammation of the pancreas.

PARALYSIS (pah-RAL-ih-sis):   loss or impairment of movement in a part of the body.

PARATHYROID GLANDS (par-ah-THI-royd glanz):   four endocrine glands behind the thyroid gland. These glands are concerned with maintaining the proper levels of calcium in the blood and bones.

PATELLA (pah-TEL-ah):   knee cap.

PATHOLOGIST (pah-THOL-o-jist):   specialist in the study of disease, by examination of tissues and cells. A pathologist examines biopsy samples and performs autopsies.

PATHOLOGY (pah-THOL-o-je):   study of disease.

PEDIATRICIAN (pe-de-ah-TRISH-un):   specialist in the treatment of childhood diseases.

PEDIATRICS (pe-de-AT-riks):   branch of medicine specializing in the treatment of diseases in children.

PELVIC (PEL-vik):   pertaining to the hip bone (pelvis) or region of the hip.

PELVIC CAVITY (PEL-vik KAV-ih-te):   space contained within the hip bone (front and sides) and the lower part of the backbone (sacrum and coccyx). The urinary bladder and the uterus (in females) are organs within the pelvic cavity.

PELVIS (PEL-vis):   hip bone. The pelvis is composed of the ilium (upper portion), ischium (lower portion), and the pubis (front portion).

PENICILLIN (pen-ih-SIL-in):   substance, derived from certain molds (fungi), that can destroy bacteria; an antibiotic.

PENIS (PE-nis):   external male organ containing the urethra, through which both urine and semen (sperm cells and fluid) leave the body.

PEPTIC ULCER (PEP-tik UL-ser): sore (lesion) of the mucous membrane lining the first part of the small intestine or stomach.

PERCUTANEOUS (per-ku-TAN-e-us): pertaining to through the skin.

PERIANAL (per-e-A-nal): pertaining to surrounding the ANUS.

PERIOSTEUM (per-e-OS-te-um): membrane that surrounds bone.

PERITONEAL (per-ih-to-NE-al): pertaining to the PERITONEUM.

PERITONEAL DIALYSIS: (per-i-to-NE-al di-AL-ih-sis): process of removing wastes from the blood by introducing a special fluid into the ABDOMEN. The wastes seep into the fluid from the bloodstream, and then the fluid is drained from the body.

PERITONEOSCOPY (per-ih-to-ne-OS-ko-pe): process of viewing the peritoneum. A small incision is made near the navel, and an instrument (peritoneoscope) is inserted to view the organs within the peritoneum. Also called LAPAROSCOPY.

PERITONEUM (per-ih-to-NE-um): membrane that surrounds the abdomen and holds the abdominal organs in place.

PHALANGES (fah-LAN-jez): finger bones.

PHARYNGEAL (fah-rin-JE-al): pertaining to the pharynx (throat).

PHARYNGITIS (fah-rin-JI-tis): inflammation of the pharynx (throat).

PHARYNX (FAR-inks): The organ behind the mouth that receives swallowed food and delivers it to the esophagus. The pharynx also receives air from the nose and passes it to the trachea (windpipe). Also known as the throat.

PHLEBOTOMY (fle-BOT-o-me): incision of a vein.

PHRENIC (FREH-nik): pertaining to the diaphragm.

PHYSICAL MEDICINE AND REHABILITATION (FIZ-e-kal MED-i-sin and re-ha-bil-i-TA-shun): field of medicine that specializes in restoring the function of the body after illness.

PINEAL GLAND (pi-NE-al gland): small gland within the brain that secretes a hormone, melatonin. Its exact function is unclear. In lower animals, the pineal gland is a receptor of light.

PITUITARY GLAND (pi-TU-i-tar-e gland): organ at the base of the brain that secretes many different hormones. These hormones enter the blood to regulate other organs and endocrine glands. For example, growth hormone from the pituitary gland affects the growth of bones, thyroid-stimulating hormone controls the thyroid gland, and follicle-stimulating hormone affects the ovaries.

PLATELET (PLAT-let): cell in the blood that aids clotting; thrombocyte.

PLEURA (PLUR-ah): double membrane that surrounds the lungs.

PLEURAL EFFUSION (PLUR-al e-FU-zhun): collection of fluid between the double membrane that surrounds the lungs.

PLEURISY (PLU-rih-se): inflammation of the PLEURA.

PLEURITIS (plu-RI-tis): inflammation of the PLEURA.

PNEUMONIA (nu-MO-ne-ah): abnormal condition of the lungs (PNEUMON/O), marked by inflammation and collection of material within the air sacs of the lungs.

PNEUMONITIS (nu-mo-NI-tis): inflammation of a lung or lungs.

PNEUMOTHORAX (nu-mo-THO-raks):   abnormal accumulation of air in the space between the pleura.

POLYDIPSIA (pol-e-DIP-se-ah):   excessive (POLY-) thirst (-DIPSIA).

POLYURIA (pol-e-UR-e-ah):   excessive (POLY-) urination (-URIA).

POST MORTEM (post MOR-tem):   after death.

POST PARTUM (post PAR-tum):   after birth.

POSTERIOR (pos-TER-e-or):   located in the back portion of a structure or of the body.

PRECANCEROUS (pre-KAN-ser-us):   pertaining to a condition that may come before a cancer; a condition that tends to become malignant.

PRENATAL (pre-NA-tal):   pertaining to before birth.

PROCTOLOGIST (prok-TOL-o-jist):   medical doctor who specializes in study of the anus and rectum.

PROGNOSIS (prog-NO-sis):   forecast as to the probable outcome of an illness or treatment; literally, before (PRO-) knowledge (-GNOSIS).

PROLAPSE (pro-LAPS):   falling down, drooping of a part of the body; literally, a sliding (-LAPSE) forward (PRO-).

PROSTATE GLAND (PROS-tat gland):   male gland that surrounds the base of the urinary bladder. It produces fluid that leaves the body with sperm cells.

PROSTATECTOMY (pros-ta-TEK-to-me):   removal (excision) of the prostate gland.

PROSTATIC (pros-TAH-tik):   pertaining to the prostate gland.

PROSTHESIS (pros-THE-sis):   artificial substitute for a missing part of the body; literally, to place (-THESIS) before (PROS-).

PROTEINURIA (pro-ten-U-re-ah):   abnormal condition of protein in the urine; albuminuria.

PSYCHIATRIST (si-KI-ah-trist):   specialist in treatment of the mind and mental disorders.

PSYCHIATRY (si-KI-ah-tre):   treatment of disorders of the mind.

PSYCHOLOGY (si-KOL-o-je):   study of the mind.

PSYCHOSIS (si-KO-sis):   abnormal condition of the mind; serious mental disorder that involves loss of normal perception of reality.

PULMONARY (PUL-mo-ner-e):   pertaining to the lungs.

PULMONARY CIRCULATION (PUL-mon-ner-e ser-ku-LA-shun):   passage of blood from the heart to the lungs and back to the heart.

PULMONARY EDEMA (PUL-mon-ner-e eh-DE-mah):   abnormal collection of fluid in the lung (within the air sacs of the lung).

PULMONARY SPECIALIST (PUL-mo-ner-e SPESH-ah-list):   specialist in treatment of lung disorders.

PUPIL (PU-pil):   black center of the eye through which light enters.

PYELITIS (pi-eh-LI-tis):   inflammation of the renal pelvis.

RADIOLOGIST (ra-de-OL-o-jist):   specialist in the use of x-rays to diagnose illness. A radiologist also uses ultrasound and magnetic resonance imaging techniques.

RADIOLOGY (ra-de-OL-o-je):   science of using x-rays in the diagnosis of disease.

RADIOTHERAPIST (ra-de-o-THER-ah-pist):   specialist in treatment of disease using high-energy x-rays.

RADIOTHERAPY (ra-de-o-THER-ah-pe):   treatment of disease using high-energy x-rays.

RADIUS (RA-de-us):   one of two lower arm bones, the one on the thumb side of the hand.

RECTAL RESECTION (REK-tal re-SEK-shun):   excision (resection) of the rectum.

RECTOCELE (REK-to-sel):   hernia (protrusion) of the rectum into the vagina.

RECTUM (REK-tum):   end of the colon; delivers wastes (feces) to the anus.

RELAPSE (re-LAPS):   return of disease after it appeared to stop.

REMISSION (re-MISH-un):   lessening of symptoms of a disease.

RENAL (RE-nal):   pertaining to the kidney.

RENAL FAILURE (RE-nal FAL-ur):   kidneys stop functioning.

RENAL PELVIS (RE-nal PEL-vis):   central section of the kidney.

RESEARCH (RE-surch):   laboratory investigation of a medical problem.

RESECTION (re-SEK-shun):   removal (excision) of an organ or structure.

RESIDENCY TRAINING (RES-i-den-se TRAY-ning):   period of hospital work involving care of patients after completion of four years of medical school.

RESPIRATORY SYSTEM (RES-pir-ah-tor-e SIS-tem):   organs that control breathing, allowing air to enter and leave the body.

RETINA (RET-ih-nah):   layer of sensitive cells at the back of the eye. Light is focused on the retina and is then transmitted to the optic nerve, which leads to the brain.

RETINOPATHY (reh-tin-OP-a-the):   disease of the RETINA.

RETROGASTRIC (reh-tro-GAS-trik):   pertaining to behind the stomach.

RETROPERITONEAL (reh-tro-per-ih-to-NE-al):   pertaining to behind the peritoneum.

RHEUMATOID ARTHRITIS (RU-mah-toyd arth-RI-tis):   chronic inflammatory disease of joints and connective tissue leading to deformed joints.

RHEUMATOLOGIST (ru-mah-TOL-o-jist):   specialist in treatment of diseases of joints and muscles. RHEUMAT/O comes from the Greek *rheuma,* meaning "that which flows, as a stream or a river." Inflammatory disorders of joints and various forms of arthritis are marked by a collection of fluid in the joint space.

RHEUMATOLOGY (ru-mah-TOL-o-je):   study of joint and muscle diseases.

RHINITIS (ri-NI-tis):   inflammation of the nose.

RHINOPLASTY (RI-no-plas-te):   surgical repair of the nose.

RHINORRHEA (ri-no-RE-ah):   discharge (-RRHEA) from the nose (RHIN/O).

RHINOTOMY (ri-NOT-o-me):   incision of the nose.

RIB (rib):   one of twelve paired bones surrounding the chest. Seven ribs (true ribs) attach directly to the breastbone, three (false ribs) attach to the seventh rib, and two (floating ribs) are not attached at all.

SACRAL (SA-kral):   pertaining to the sacrum (the triangular bone just below the lumbar vertebrae in the back).

SACRAL REGION (SA-kral RE-jin): five fused bones in the lower back, below the lumbar bones and wedged between two parts of the hip (ilium).

SACRUM (SA-krum): triangular bone in the lower back just below the lumbar bones and formed by five fused bones.

SAGITTAL PLANE (SAJ-ih-tal plan): an imaginary line that divides an organ or the body into a right and a left portion.

SAGITTAL SECTION (SAJ-ih-tal SEK-shun): a cut (section) through the body dividing it into right and left parts.

SALPINGECTOMY (sal-pin-JEK-to-me): removal of a fallopian (uterine) tube.

SALPINGITIS (sal-pin-JI-tis): inflammation of a fallopian (uterine) tube.

SARCOMA (sar-KO-mah): cancerous tumor of connective (flesh) tissue, such as bone, muscle, fat, or cartilage.

SCAPULA (SKAP-u-lah): shoulder bone.

SCLERA (SKLE-rah): white, outer coat of the eyeball.

SCROTAL (SKRO-tal): pertaining to the scrotum.

SCROTUM (SKRO-tum): sac on the outside of the body that contains the testes.

SEBACEOUS GLAND (seh-BA-shus gland): oil (sebum)-producing gland in the skin.

SECTION (SEK-shun): an act of cutting.

SELLA TURCICA (SEL-ah TUR-sih-ka): cup-like depression in the base of the skull that holds the pituitary gland.

SEMEN (SE-men): fluid composed of sperm cells and secretions from the prostate and other glands in the male.

SENSE ORGANS (sens OR-ganz): parts of the body that receive messages from the environment and relay them to the brain so that we see, hear, and feel sensations. Examples of sense organs are the eye, ear, and skin.

SEPTIC (SEP-tik): pertaining to infection.

SEPTICEMIA (sep-ti-SE-me-ah): condition of infection in the blood. Septicemia is commonly called blood poisoning and is associated with the presence of bacteria or their poisons in the blood.

SHOCK (shok): group of symptoms (pale skin, rapid pulse, shallow breathing) that indicate poor oxygen supply to tissue and insufficient return of blood to the heart.

SIGMOID COLON (SIG-moyd KO-len): S-shaped lower portion of the colon.

SKIN (skin): outer covering that protects the body.

SKULL (skul): bone that surrounds the brain and the other organs in the head.

SMALL INTESTINE (smal in-TES-tin): organ that receives food from the stomach; it is divided into three sections—duodenum, jejunum, and ileum.

SONOGRAM (SON-o-gram): record of sound waves after they bounce off organs in the body; also called *ultrasound exam* or *echogram.*

SPINAL CAVITY (SPI-nal KAV-ih-te): space in the back that contains the spinal cord and is surrounded by the backbones.

SPINAL COLUMN (SPI-nal KOL-um): backbones; vertebrae.

SPINAL CORD (SPI-nal kord): bundle of nerves that extends from the brain down the back and is surrounded by backbones. The spinal cord carries electrical messages to and from the brain.

SPINAL NERVES (SPI-nal nervz):   nerves that transmit messages to and from the spinal cord.

SPLEEN (splen):   organ in the upper left abdomen that stores blood cells. It also destroys red blood cells, setting free the hemoglobin that is in the cells, and produces white blood cells, called *lymphocytes.*

SPLENOMEGALY (splehn-o-MEG-ah-le):   enlargement of the spleen.

SPONDYLOSIS (spon-di-LO-sis):   abnormal condition of a vertebra or vertebrae.

STERNUM (STER-num):   breast bone.

STOMACH (STUM-ak):   organ that receives food from the esophagus and sends it to the small intestine. Some digestion takes place in the stomach.

STOMATITIS (sto-mah-TI-tis):   inflammation of the mouth.

STROKE (strok):   cerebrovascular accident. Trauma to or blockage of the blood vessels within the brain leads to less blood supply to brain tissue. This causes cells to die and loss of function to the part of the body controlled by those nerve cells.

SUBCOSTAL (sub-KOS-tal):   pertaining to below the ribs.

SUBCUTANEOUS (sub-ku-TA-ne-us):   pertaining to below the skin.

SUBCUTANEOUS TISSUE (sub-ku-TA-ne-us TIS-u):   lower layer of the skin composed of fatty tissue.

SUBDURAL HEMATOMA (sub-DUR-al he-mah-TO-mah):   collection of blood under the dura mater (outermost layer of the membranes surrounding the brain).

SUBGASTRIC (sub-GAS-trik):   pertaining to below the stomach.

SUBHEPATIC (sub-heh-PAT-ik):   pertaining to under the liver.

SUBSCAPULAR (sub-SKAP-u-lar):   pertaining to under the shoulder bone.

SUBTOTAL (sub-TO-tal):   less than total; just under the total amount.

SURGERY (SUR-jer-e):   branch of medicine that treats disease by manual (hand) or operative methods.

SWEAT GLAND (sweht gland):   gland in the skin that produces a watery substance containing salts.

SYNDROME (SIN-drom):   set of symptoms and signs of disease that occur together to indicate a disease condition.

SYSTEM (SIS-tem):   group of organs working together to do a job in the body. For example, the digestive system includes the mouth, throat, stomach, and intestines, all of which help to bring food into the body, break it down, and deliver it to the bloodstream.

SYSTEMIC CIRCULATION (sis-TEM-ik ser-ku-LA-shun):   the passage of blood from the heart to the tissues of the body and back to the heart.

TACHYCARDIA (tak-eh-KAR-de-ah):   condition of fast, rapid heartbeat.

TACHYPNEA (tak-ip-NE-ah):   condition of rapid breathing.

TENDON (TEN-don):   connective tissue that joins muscles to bones.

TESTICLE (TES-tih-kl):   see TESTIS.

TESTIS (TES-tis):   one of two paired male organs in the scrotum. The testes (pl.) produce sperm cells and male hormone; also called testicles.

THORACENTESIS (tho-rah-sen-TE-sis):   surgical puncture of the chest to remove fluid.

THORACIC (tho-RAS-ik):   pertaining to the chest.

THORACIC CAVITY (tho-RAS-ik KAV-ih-te):   space above the abdomen, containing the heart, lungs, and other organs; the chest cavity.

THORACIC REGION (tho-RAS-ik RE-jun):   backbones that are attached to the ribs. These bones are below the cervical bones and above the lumbar bones.

THORACIC SURGEON (tho-RAS-ik SUR-jin):   doctor who operates on organs in the chest.

THORACIC VERTEBRA (tho-RAS-ik VER-te-brah):   a backbone in the chest.

THORACOCENTESIS (tho-rah-ko-sen-TE-sis):   surgical puncture to remove fluid from the chest; thoracentesis.

THORACOTOMY (tho-rah-KOT-o-me):   incision of the chest.

THROAT (throt):   see PHARYNX.

THROMBOCYTE (THROM-bo-sīt):   clotting cell; a platelet.

THROMBOSIS (throm-BO-sis):   abnormal condition of clot formation.

THROMBUS (THROM-bus):   blood clot.

THYMOMA (thi-MO-mah):   tumor of the thymus gland.

THYMUS GLAND (THI-mus gland):   endocrine gland in the middle of the chest that produces a hormone, thymosin. A much larger gland in children, it is believed that the thymus aids the immune system by stimulating the production of white blood cells.

THYROADENITIS (thi-ro-ah-de-NI-tis):   inflammation of the thyroid gland.

THYROID GLAND (THI-royd gland):   endocrine gland in the neck that produces hormones that act on cells all over the body. The hormone increases the activity of cells by stimulating the production of energy.

THYROXINE (thi-ROK-sin):   hormone secreted by the thyroid gland; also known as T_4.

TIBIA (TIB-e-ah):   larger of the two lower leg bones; the shin bone.

TISSUE (TISH-u):   groups of similar cells that work together to do a job in the body; muscle tissue, nerve tissue, and epithelial (skin) tissue.

TISSUE CAPILLARIES (TISH-u KAP-ih-lar-ez):   tiny blood vessels that lie near cells and through whose walls gases, food, and waste materials pass.

TOMOGRAPHY (to-MOG-rah-fe):   series of x-ray pictures that show an organ in depth, as if to see "slices" of an organ.

TONSILLECTOMY (ton-si-LEK-to-me):   removal (excision) of a tonsil or tonsils.

TONSILS (TON-silz):   lymphatic tissue in back of the mouth near the throat.

TRACHEA (TRAY-ke-ah):   tube that carries air from the throat to the BRONCHIAL TUBES; windpipe.

TRACHEOSTOMY (tray-ke-OS-to-me):   opening of the windpipe to the outside of the body.

TRACHEOTOMY (tray-ke-OT-o-me):   incision of the trachea.

TRANSABDOMINAL (trans-ab-DOM-ih-nal):   pertaining to across the abdomen.

TRANSGASTRIC (trans-GAS-trik):   pertaining to across the stomach.

TRANSURETHRAL (trans-u-RE-thral):   pertaining to across (through) the urethra. A transurethral prostatectomy is removal of the prostate gland by surgery through the urethra.

TRANSVERSE PLANE (trans-VERS plan):   imaginary line that divides an organ or the body into an upper and lower portion; a cross-sectional plane.

TRICUSPID VALVE (tri-KUS-pid valv):   valve on the right side of the heart that separates the upper right chamber (ATRIUM) from the lower right chamber (VENTRICLE). It has three (TRI-) cusps or points.

TYMPANIC MEMBRANE (tim-PAN-ik MEM-bran):   see EARDRUM.

TYMPANOPLASTY   (tim-pan-o-PLAS-te): surgical   repair   of   the   eardrum (TYMPAN/O).

ULCER (UL-ser):   sore or defect in the surface of an organ which is produced by destruction of tissue.

ULNA (UL-nah):   one of two lower arm bones, the one on the little finger side of the hand.

ULTRASONOGRAPHY (ul-tra-son-OG-rah-fe):   recording internal body structure using sound waves.

ULTRASOUND (UL-tra-sownd):   sound waves with greater frequency than can be heard by the human ear. This energy is used to detect abnormalities by beaming the waves into the body and recording the echoes that reflect off tissues.

UNILATERAL (u-nih-LAT-er-al):   pertaining to one side.

UREA (u-RE-ah):   chief nitrogen-containing waste that the kidney removes from the blood and eliminates from the body in urine.

UREMIA (u-RE-me-ah):   abnormal condition of excessive amounts of the waste material urea in the bloodstream.

URETER (u-RE-ter):   one of two tubes that lead from the kidney to the bladder.

URETERECTOMY (u-re-ter-EK-to-me):   removal (excision) of a ureter.

URETHRA (u-RE-thrah):   tube that carries urine from the bladder to the outside of the body. In males, the urethra, which is within the penis, also carries sperm from the vas deferens to the outside of the body when sperm is discharged (ejaculation).

URETHRAL STRICTURE (u-RE-thral STRIK-shur):   narrowing of the urethra.

URETHRITIS (u-re-THRI-tis):   inflammation of the urethra.

URINALYSIS (u-rih-NAL-ih-sis):   examination of urine to determine its contents.

URINARY BLADDER (UR-in-er-e BLA-der):   muscular sac that holds urine and then releases it to leave the body through the urethra.

URINARY SYSTEM (UR-in-er-e SIS-tem):   organs that produce and send urine out of the body. These organs are the kidneys, ureters, bladder, and urethra.

URINARY TRACT (UR-in-er-e trakt):   tubes that carry urine from the kidney to the outside of the body.

URINE (UR-in):   fluid that is produced by the kidneys, passed through the ureters, stored in the bladder, and released from the body through the urethra.

UROLOGIST (u-ROL-o-jist):   specialist in operating on the urinary tract in males and females and the reproductive tract in males.

UROLOGY (u-ROL-o-je):   study of the urinary system in males and females and the reproductive tract in males.

UTERINE (U-ter-in):   pertaining to the uterus.

UTERINE TUBES (U-ter-in tubz):   see FALLOPIAN TUBES.

UTERUS (U-ter-us):   muscular organ in a female that holds and provides nourishment for the developing fetus; womb.

VAGINA (vah-JI-nah):   muscular passageway from the uterus to the outside of the body.

VAGINITIS (vah-ji-NI-tis):   inflammation of the vagina.

VAS DEFERENS (vas DEHF-er-enz):   one of two tubes that carry sperm from the testes to the urethra.

VASCULAR (VAS-ku-lar):   pertaining to blood vessels.

VASCULITIS (vas-ku-LI-tis):   inflammation of blood vessels.

VASECTOMY (vas-EK-to-me):   removal (excision) of a part of the vas deferens so that sperm cells are prevented from becoming part of semen.

VASOCONSTRICTOR (vas-o-kon-STRIK-tor):   drug that narrows blood vessels, especially small arteries.

VEIN (van):   blood vessel that carries blood back to the heart from the tissues of the body.

VENTRICLE (VEN-tri-kl):   one of the two lower chambers of the heart. The right ventricle receives blood from the right atrium (upper chamber) and sends it to the lungs. The left ventricle receives blood from the left atrium and sends it to the body through the aorta.

VENULE (VEN-ul):   small vein.

VENULITIS (ven-u-LI-tis):   inflammation of a small vein.

VERTEBRA (VER-teh-brah):   backbone.

VERTEBRAE (VER-teh-bray):   backbones.

VERTEBRAL (VER-teh-bral):   pertaining to a backbone.

VESICAL (VES-i-kal):   pertaining to the urinary bladder (VESIC/O).

VIRUS (VI-rus):   small infectious agent that can reproduce itself only when it is inside another living cell.

WOMB (woom):   see UTERUS.

GLOSSARY OF WORD PARTS

Section I of this glossary is a list of **medical terminology** word parts and their **English** meanings. Section II is the reverse of that list, giving **English** meanings and their corresponding **medical terminology** word parts.

SECTION I: MEDICAL TERMINOLOGY → ENGLISH

Word Part	Meaning
a-, an-	no, not
ab-	away from
abdomin/o	abdomen
-ac	pertaining to
ad-	toward
aden/o	gland
adren/o	adrenal gland
-al	pertaining to
-algia	pain
alveol/o	alveolus (air sac within the lung)
amni/o	amnion (sac that surrounds the embryo)
-an	pertaining to
ana-	up, apart
an/o	anus
angi/o	vessel (blood)
ante-	before, forward
anti-	against
append/o, appendic/o	appendix
-ar	pertaining to
arteri/o	artery
arteriol/o	small artery
arthr/o	joint
-ary	pertaining to
-ation	process, condition
axill/o	armpit
balan/o	penis
bi-	two
bi/o	life
brady-	slow
bronch/o	bronchial tube
bronchiol/o	small bronchial tube
capillar/o	capillary
carcin/o	cancer, cancerous
cardi/o	heart
carp/o	wrist bones
-cele	hernia
-centesis	surgical puncture to remove fluid
cephal/o	head

cerebell/o	cerebellum (part of the brain)
cerebr/o	cerebrum (largest part of the brain)
cervic/o	neck
chem/o	drug, chemical
cholecyst/o	gallbladder
choledoch/o	common bile duct
chondr/o	cartilage
chron/o	time
-cision	process of cutting
cis/o	to cut
-coccus	berry-shaped bacteria (pl. cocci)
coccyg/o	tailbone
col/o	colon (large intestine)
colon/o	colon
colp/o	vagina
con-	with, together
-coniosis	dust
coron/o	heart
cost/o	rib
crani/o	skull
crin/o	secrete
-crine	secretion
-crit	separate
cutane/o	skin
cyst/o	urinary bladder
cyt/o	cell
-cyte	cell
dermat/o, derm/o	skin
dia-	through, complete
dur/o	dura mater
dys-	bad, painful, difficult
-eal	pertaining to
ec-	out, outside
ecto-	out, outside
-ectomy	excision (resection, removal)
-emesis	vomiting
-emia	blood condition
en-	within, in, inner
encephal/o	brain
endo-	within, in, inner
endocrin/o,	endocrine glands
endometr/o	endometrium (inner lining of the uterus)
enter/o	intestines (usually small intestine)
epi-	above, upon
epiglott/o	epiglottis
epitheli/o	skin (surface tissue)

erythr/o	red
esophag/o	esophagus
esthesi/o	sensation
ex-, extra-	out, outside
gastr/o	stomach
gen/o	to produce
-gen	to produce
-genesis	producing, forming
-genic	pertaining to producing, produced by
ger/o	old age
glyc/o	sugar
gnos/o	knowledge
-gram	record
-graphy	process of recording, to record
gynec/o	woman, female
hemat/o, hem/o	blood
hepat/o	liver
hyper-	excessive, above
hypo-	below, deficient
hypophys/o	pituitary gland
hyster/o	uterus
-ia	condition
iatr/o	treatment
-ic	pertaining to
in-	in, into
-ine	pertaining to
inguin/o	groin
inter-	between
intra-	within
isch/o	to hold back
-ism	condition
-ist	specialist
-itis	inflammation
lapar/o	abdomen
laryng/o	larynx (voice box)
later/o	side
leuk/o	white
-listhesis	to slip, slide
lith/o	stone
-lith	stone
-logy	study of
lumb/o	loin, waist region
lymph/o	lymph
lymphaden/o	lymph nodes
lymphangi/o	lymph vessel
lys/o	separation, breakdown, destruction

-lysis	separation, breakdown, destruction
mal-	bad
mamm/o	breast
mast/o	breast
mediastin/o	mediastinum
-megaly	enlargement
men/o	menstruation
mening/o	meninges (membranes covering brain and spinal cord)
meta-	beyond
metr/o	uterus; to measure
-metry	measurement
-mortem	death
-motor	movement
muscul/o	muscle
my/o	muscle
myel/o	bone marrow (with -blast, -oma, -cyte, -genic)
myel/o	spinal cord (with -algia, -gram, -itis, -cele)
myos/o	muscle
myring/o	eardrum
nas/o	nose
nat/i	birth
neo-	new
nephr/o	kidney
neur/o	nerve
obstetr/o	midwife
ocul/o	eye
-oma	tumor, mass, swelling
onc/o	tumor
oophor/o	ovary
ophthalm/o	eye
-opsy	process of viewing
opt/o	eye
or/o	mouth
orch/o	testicle
orchid/o	testicle
orth/o	straight
-osis	abnormal condition
oste/o	bone
ot/o	ear
-ous	pertaining to
ovari/o	ovary
pancreat/o	pancreas
para-	near, along the side of
-partum	birth

path/o	disease
-pathy	disease condition
ped/o	child
pelv/o	hip bone
per-	through
peri-	surrounding
peritone/o	peritoneum (membrane around abdominal organs)
-pexy	fixation (surgical)
pharyng/o	pharynx, throat
-philia	attraction to
phleb/o	vein
phren/o	diaphragm
phren/o	mind
plas/o	formation, growth, development
-plasm	formation, growth, development
-plasty	surgical repair
-plegia	paralysis
pleur/o	pleura (membranes surrounding the lungs)
-pnea	breathing
pneum/o	air, lung
pneumon/o	lung
-poiesis	formation
post-	after, behind
pre-	before
pro-, pros-	before, forward
proct/o	anus and rectum
prostat/o	prostate gland
psych/o	mind
-ptosis	prolapse, sagging
-ptysis	spitting
pulmon/o	lung
pyel/o	renal pelvis (central section of the kidney)
radi/o	x-ray
re-, retro-	behind, back
rect/o	rectum
ren/o	kidney
retin/o	retina of the eye
rheumat/o	flow, fluid
rhin/o	nose
-rrhage	bursting forth of blood
-rrhagia	bursting forth of blood
-rrhea	flow, discharge
sacr/o	sacrum
salping/o	fallopian (uterine) tube, eustachian tube
-salpinx	fallopian (uterine) tube, eustachian tube

sarc/o	flesh
scapul/o	shoulder blade (bone)
-sclerosis	condition of hardening
-scope	instrument to view or visually examine
-scopy	process of viewing or visual examination
scrot/o	scrotal sac, scrotum
-section	to cut
-sept/o	infection
septic/o	infection
-sis	condition
-somatic	pertaining to the body
son/o	sound
-spasm	constriction
spin/o	backbone
splen/o	spleen
spondyl/o	vertebra, backbone
-stasis	stop, control
-stat	stop, control
-stomy	opening
sub-	under, below
sym-	with, together (use before b, p, and m)
syn-	with, together
tachy-	fast
-tension	pressure
-therapy	treatment
-thesis	to put or place
thorac/o	chest
thromb/o	clot
thym/o	thymus gland
thyr/o, thyroid/o	thyroid gland
-tic	pertaining to
-tomy	incision, cut into
tonsill/o	tonsils
top/o	to put, place
trache/o	trachea (windpipe)
trans-	across, through
tri-	three
troph/o	development, nourishment
-trophy	development, nourishment
tympan/o	eardrum
ultra-	beyond
-um	structure
uni-	one
ureter/o	ureter
urethr/o	urethra
ur/o	urine, urinary tract

-uria	urine condition
uter/o	uterus
vagin/o	vagina
vas/o	vessel, vas deferens
vascul/o	blood vessel
ven/o	vein
vertebr/o	vertebra (backbone)
vesic/o	urinary bladder

SECTION II: ENGLISH → MEDICAL TERMINOLOGY

Meaning	Word Part
abdomen	abdomin/o (use with -al, -centesis)
	lapar/o (use with -scope, -scopy, -tomy)
abnormal condition	-osis
above	epi-, hyper-
across	trans-
adrenal gland	adren/o
after	post-
against	anti-
air	pneum/o
air sac	alveol/o
along the side of	para-
alveolus	alveol/o
amnion	amni/o
anus	an/o
anus and rectum	proct/o
apart	ana-
appendix	append/o (use with -ectomy)
	appendic/o (use with -itis)
armpit	axill/o
artery	arteri/o
attraction to	-philia
away from	ab-
backbone	spin/o (use with -al)
	spondyl/o (use with -itis, -listhesis, -osis, -pathy)
	vertebr/o (use with -al)
bacteria (berry-shaped)	-coccus (pl. -cocci)
bad	dys-, mal-
before	ante-, pre-, pro-, pros-
behind	post-, re-, retro-
below	hypo-, sub-
between	inter-

beyond	meta-, ultra-
birth	nat/i, -partum
bladder (urinary)	cyst/o (use with -ic, -itis, -cele, -gram, -scopy)
	vesic/o (use with -al, -stomy, -tomy)
blood	hem/o (use with -cyte, -dialysis, -globin, -lysis, -philia, -ptysis, -rrhage, -stasis, -stat)
	hemat/o (use with -crit, -emesis, -logist, -logy, -oma, -poiesis, -salpinx, -uria)
blood condition	-emia
blood vessel	angi/o (use with -ectomy, -dysplasia, -genesis, -gram, -graphy, -oma, -plasty, -spasm)
	vas/o (use with -constriction, -dilatation, -motor)
	vascul/o (use with -ar, -itis)
body	-somatic
bone	oste/o
bone marrow	myel/o
brain	encephal/o
breakdown	-lysis, lys/o
breast	mamm/o (use with -ary, -gram, -graphy, -plasty)
	mast/o (use with -algia, -ectomy, -itis)
breathing	-pnea
bronchial tube	bronch/o
bronchiole	bronchiol/o
bursting forth of blood	-rrhage, -rrhagia
cancer	carcin/o
cancerous	carcin/o
capillary	capillar/o
cartilage	chondr/o
cell	-cyte, cyt/o
cerebellum	cerebell/o
cerebrum	cerebr/o
chemical	chem/o
chest	thorac/o
child	ped/o
clot	thromb/o
colon	col/o (use with -ectomy, -itis, -stomy)
	colon/o (use with -pathy, -scope, -scopy)
common bile duct	choledoch/o
complete	dia-
condition	-ation, -ia, -ism, -osis, -sis, -y
constriction	-spasm
control	-stasis, -stat

cut	-cision, cis/o, -section, -tomy
death	-mortem, necr/o
deficient	hypo-
destroy	lys/o, -lysis
development	troph/o, -trophy
diaphragm	phren/o
difficult	dys-
discharge	-rrhea
disease	path/o, -pathy
drug	chem/o
dura mater	dur/o
dust	-coniosis
ear	ot/o
eardrum	myring/o (use with -ectomy, -itis, -tomy)
	tympan/o (use with -ic, -metry, -plasty)
electricity	electr/o
endocrine gland	endocrin/o
endometrium	endometr/o
enlargement	-megaly
epiglottis	epiglott/o
esophagus	esophag/o
eustachian tube	salping/o
excessive	hyper-
eye	ocul/o (use with -ar, -facial, -motor)
	ophthalm/o (use with -ia, -ic, -logist, -logy, -pathy, -plasty, -plegia, -scope, -scopy)
	opt/o (use with -ic, -metrist)
fallopian tube	salping/o, -salpinx
fast	tachy-
female	gynec/o
fixation (surgical)	-pexy
flesh	sarc/o
flow	-rrhea
fluid	rheumat/o
formation	plas/o, -plasm, -poiesis, -genesis
forward	ante-, pro-, pros-
gallbladder	cholecyst/o
gland	aden/o
groin	inguin/o
growth	plas/o, -plasm
hardening	-sclerosis
head	cephal/o
heart	cardi/o (use with -ac, -graphy, -logy, -logist, -megaly, -pathy, -vascular)
	coron/o (use with -ary)
hernia	-cele

hip bone	pelv/o
hold back	isch/o
in, into	in-, en-
incision	-tomy, -section
infection	sept/o, septic/o
inflammation	-itis
inner	endo-
instrument to record	-graph
instrument to view	-scope
intestines	enter/o
joint	arthr/o
kidney	nephr/o (use with -algia, -ectomy, -ic, -itis, -lith, -megaly, -oma, -osis, -pathy, -ptosis, -sclerosis, -stomy, -tomy)
	ren/o (use with -al, -gram)
kidney (central section)	pyel/o
knowledge	gnos/o
larynx	laryng/o
life	bi/o
liver	hepat/o
loin	lumb/o
lung	pneum/o (use with -coccus, -coniosis)
	pneumon/o (use with -ectomy, -ia, -ic, -itis, -pathy, -therapy, -thorax)
	pulmon/o (use with -ary)
lymph	lymph/o
lymph node	lymphaden/o
lymph vessel	lymphangi/o
mass	-oma
measure	metr/o, -meter, -metry
mediastinum	mediastin/o
meninges	mening/o
menstruation	men/o
midwife	obstetr/o
mind	psych/o
mouth	or/o (use with -al)
	stomat/o (use with -itis)
movement	-motor
muscle	muscul/o (use with -ar, -skeletal)
	myos/o (use with -itis)
	my/o (use with -ectomy, -oma, -gram, -neural)
near	para-
neck	cervic/o
nerve	neur/o
new	neo-

no, not	a-, an-
nose	nas/o (use with -al)
	rhin/o (use with -itis, -rrhea, -plasty)
nourishment	troph/o, -trophy
old age	ger/o
one	uni-
opening	-stomy
out, outside	ec-, ecto-, ex-, extra-
ovary	oophor/o (use with -cyte, -itis, -ectomy, -plasty, -tomy)
	ovari/o (use with -an)
pain	-algia
pancreas	pancreat/o
paralysis	-plegia
pelvis	pelv/o
pelvis (renal)	pyel/o
penis	balan/o
peritoneum	peritone/o
pertaining to	-ac, -al, -an, -ar, -ary, -eal, -ic, -ine, -ous, -tic
pharynx	pharyng/o
pituitary gland	hypophys/o
pleura	pleur/o
pressure	-tension
process	-ation, -ism
process of cutting	-cision, -tomy, -section
process of recording	-graphy
process of viewing	-opsy, -scopy
produce (to)	-gen, gen/o
produced by	-genic
producing	-genic, -genesis
prolapse	-ptosis
prostate gland	prostat/o
puncture to remove fluid	-centesis
put, place	top/o, -thesis
record	-gram
recording (process)	-graphy
rectum	rect/o
red	erythr/o
repair	-plasty
retina	retin/o
rib	cost/o
sacrum	sacr/o
sagging	-ptosis
scapula	scapul/o
scrotum	scrot/o
secrete, secretion	-crine, crin/o

sensation	esthesi/o
separation	-crit, -lysis
shoulder blade	scapul/o
side	later/o
skin	cutane/o (use with -ous)
	derm/o, dermat/o (use with -itis, -logy, -osis)
	epitheli/o (use with -al)
skull	crani/o
slip (to)	-listhesis
slow	brady-
small artery	arteri/o
small intestine	enter/o
sound	son/o
specialist	-ist
spinal cord	myel/o
spine	spin/o
spitting	-ptysis
spleen	splen/o
stomach	gastr/o
stone	lith/o, -lith
stop	-stasis, -stat
straight	orth/o
structure	-um
study of	-logy
sugar	glyc/o
surgical puncture to remove fluid	-centesis
surgical repair	-plasty
surrounding	peri-
swelling	-oma
tailbone	coccyg/o
testicle, testis	orch/o, orchi/o, orchid/o
throat	pharyng/o
three	tri-
through	dia-, per-, trans-
thymus gland	thym/o
thyroid gland	thyr/o, thyroid/o
time	chron/o
together	con-, syn-
tonsil	tonsill/o
trachea	trache/o
treatment	iatr/o, -therapy
tumor	onc/o, -oma
two	bi-
under	hypo-, sub-
up	ana-

upon	epi-
ureter	ureter/o
urethra	urethr/o
urinary bladder	cyst/o, vesic/o
urinary tract	ur/o
urine	ur/o
urine condition	-uria
uterine tube	salping/o
uterus	hyster/o (use with -ectomy, -graphy, -gram)
	metr/o (use with -itis, -rrhagia)
	uter/o (use with -ine)
uterus (inner lining)	endometri/o
vagina	colp/o (use with -pexy, -plasty, -scope, -scopy, -tomy)
	vagin/o (use with -al, -itis)
vas deferens	vas/o
vein	phleb/o (use with -ectomy, -itis, -lith, -thrombosis, -tomy)
	ven/o (use with -ous, -gram)
vertebra	spin/o (use with -al)
	spondyl/o (use with -itis, -listhesis, -osis, -pathy)
	vertebr/o (use with -al)
vessel	angi/o (use with -ectomy, -dysplasia, -genesis, -gram, -graphy, -oma, -plasty, -spasm)
	vas/o (use with -constriction, -dilatation, -motor)
	vascul/o (use with -ar, -itis)
view (to)	-opsy
visual examination	-scopy
voice box	laryng/o
waist region	lumb/o
white	leuk/o
windpipe	trache/o
with	con-, syn-
within	en-, endo-, intra-
woman	gynec/o
wrist	carp/o
x-ray	radi/o

INDEX